MAPPING
THE MIND

MAPPING THE MIND

THE SECRETS OF THE HUMAN BRAIN AND HOW IT WORKS

JOEL DAVIS

A BIRCH LANE PRESS BOOK
PUBLISHED BY CAROL PUBLISHING GROUP

A Birch Lane Press Book
Published by Carol Publishing Group
Birch Lane Press is a registered trademark of Carol Communications, Inc.

Editorial, sales and distribution, rights and permissions inquiries should be addressed to Carol Publishing Group, 120 Enterprise Avenue, Secaucus, N.J. 07094

In Canada: Canadian Manda Group, One Atlantic Avenue, Suite 105, Toronto, Ontario M6K 3E7

Carol Publishing Group books may be purchased in bulk at special discounts for sales promotion, fund-raising, or educational purposes. Special editions can be created to specifications. For details, contact Special Sales Department, 120 Enterprise Avenue, Secaucus, N.J. 07094.

Manufactured in the United States of America
10 9 8 7 6 5 4 3 2 1

Library of Congress Cataloging-in-Publication Data

Davis, Joel, 1948–
    Mapping the mind : the secrets of the human brain and how it works / Joel Davis.
        p.   cm.
    "A Birch Lane Press book."
    ISBN 1-55972-344-0 (hardcover)
    1. Brain—Popular works.   2. Neuropsychology—Popular works.
    I. Title.
QP376.D38   1996
612.8'2—dc20   95-47834
                                                                                  CIP

For Judy

CONTENTS

ACKNOWLEDGMENTS

THIS BOOK would not have been possible without the help and encouragement of many people. First, thanks go to my editors at Birch Lane Press. Hillel Black first suggested the topic of the book and then offered encouragement and support throughout the time I spent working on it. Jim Ellison shepherded the book through the editing and rewriting process with both firmness and skill. Thanks also to my agent, Joshua Bilmes, of JABberwocky Literary Agency, who has offered unflagging support during all the years he has represented me.

Many men and women in the fields of neuroscience and cognitive science and in other disciplines provided me with information, interviews, illustrations, and other support. Thanks to Marcus Raichle, Alan Gevins, Joseph LeDoux, Dean Falk, Joseph Martin, Roger Penrose, and Stephen Kosslyn for the hours of their time and, in some cases, the willingness to look over early versions of portions of the manuscript.

I am particularly grateful to the skilled hands of my two ophthalmologists, Larry Milsow in Spokane, Washington, and Edward McLean in Seattle, Washington. During the spring and summer of 1995, as I was in the middle of writing this book, I suffered a giant retinal tear in my right eye. They literally saved the sight in that eye and have worked hard to give me as much visual acuity as is currently possible.

Thanks also go to the many family members, friends, and colleagues who have supported me both during the writing of this book and the trauma of nearly losing some of my sight: my brothers, my sister, and my parents; Gene and Anne Bond, Tim and Cheryl Brinkley, Darryl Caldwell, Shirley Cannon and Devon Greyerbiehl, John and Gail Dalmas, Mary Dietzel, Tony and Ida Dolphin, Grayson Dyer, Mickey Eisenberg, Grant Meidal, Karolyn Merriman, David Murphy, Martha Norris, John and Lee Seaman, Sara Stamey, and Tom and Jan Westbrook; the librarians at the Spokane Public Library, Gonzaga University's Foley Library, the Kennedy Library at Eastern Washington

University, and the Bellingham Public Library; Judith Chander and Duane Wilkins of the University Bookstore in Seattle; the students in my "Introduction to the Nonfiction Book" class at the University of Washington; and the Community of St. Ann Church in Spokane and the members of First Presbyterian Church, in Bellingham.

I want to especially thank my parents, Gerald and Antonia Davis, for their willingness to share some of their experiences and memories with me as part of this book.

Finally, deepest thanks to my wife, Judy, without whose support I could not have written this book.

MAPPING
THE MIND

INTRODUCTION:
THE HUMAN BRAIN PROJECT

IN 1989 THE U.S. CONGRESS passed a resolution declaring the 1990s the Decade of the Brain. President George Bush signed that proclamation, and life in the world of brain research went on as usual.

Or did it?

Indeed, funding for brain research in the United States hasn't increased in any significant fashion because of the congressional proclamation. No one can point to any specific research project being carried out by any individual researcher and say, "This is being done precisely because the wise and far-seeing members of the 101st Congress proclaimed the 1990s the Decade of the Brain."

Nevertheless, this final decade of the the second millenium *is* the Decade of the Brain. Not just because of House Joint Resolution 174, though it may have played a catalytic role. It is the Decade of the Brain because neuroscientists and cognitive scientists the world over are making astonishing new discoveries about the human brain and how it works.

THE HUMAN BRAIN is the last, and greatest, scientific frontier. It is truly an internal cosmos that lies contained within our skulls. The more than 100 billion nerve cells and trillion supporting cells that make up your brain and mine constitute the most elaborate structure in the known universe. No galaxy cluster, no star, no planet, no other living creature we know of, comes even close to the brain in complexity. The number of interconnections among the brain's nerve cells is greater than the total number of atomic particles in the cosmos. Those interconnections, woven into the intricate warp and woof of the brain like some marvelous tapestry, make it possible for us to laugh, cry, rejoice, worship, create art, hate one another, love one another, learn, remember, sing, write poetry, build moon rockets, imagine impossible worlds, wish upon a star, and wonder about the nature of the brain.

1

Most brain researchers today believe that the mind itself is in some fundamental fashion a product of the brain's living activity. It is, they feel, something like a dance; it exists as long as the dancer is dancing.

Except, of course, that I can continue to watch that dance in my "mind's eye" long after the dancer and her troupe have moved on to the next city or town. One does have to be careful about some analogies, especially when talking about the brain.

For example, we're all familiar with the comparison of the brain to a computer. The brain is the body's computer. The brain is like a central processing unit with billions of little integrated chips. The brain is wetware. Careful. Careful. The brain is like a computer only in the most general sense. In most other ways that matter, it is very much unlike a computer. The most powerful computers in the world have the equivalent brainpower of a grasshopper. The confident predictions of some artificial-intelligence researchers that "computers will someday soon be thinking like humans" is far too close to hubris. For those who don't know the reference, *hubris* is an ancient Greek word meaning "excessive pride or self-confidence." In the great Greek tragedy plays, it is the hubris of the leading character—usually a powerful king—that so irritates the gods and leads them to destroy the protagonist. Artificial Intelligence wonks, beware! You don't even know *how* you *know*. That is, we have only the first real glimmerings of what the brain is doing when it is *knowing*, being self-aware, being humanly conscious. We are still a long way from the Tipperary of sentient silicon chips.

WHAT IS HAPPENING in brain research labs today is a decentralized scientific undertaking that goes by the name of the Human Brain Project. It began without benefit of congressional interest in the late 1980s as an attempt to compile the then burgeoning data about the brain. This initial attempt to create a kind of global brain database has turned into this de facto scientific project. It doesn't have a central office like the much-touted Human Genome Project (about whose origins I've written in another book). It certainly doesn't have the coordinated billion-dollar funding levels that the Human Genome Project boasts. The Human Brain Project does have at least two important factors in common with the better-known Human Genome Project: (1) smart, creative people and (2) wonderful new technology.

The people include researchers like Antonio and Hanna Damasio, Michael Davis, Wayne Drevets, Alan Gevins, Stephen Kosslyn, Joseph LeDoux, Joseph Martin, George Ojemann, Michael Posner, Marcus Raichle, Susan Schiffman, Gottfried Schlaug, and Justine Sergent.

The new technology includes machines with names like CT, MRI, PET, and SPECT. And there's also some old technology, too, such as the venerable EEG, that has been revitalized for this great scientific adventure.

The decentralized nature of the Human Brain Project could be compared to that of the Internet, the global network of computer networks. The Internet has no centralized main computer, no president or chief executive officer, no high-paid staff, and as some politicians are slowly beginning to learn, no official censor, either. It is a totally distributed network of interconnected computers and databases, all interacting with one another continually. All constantly growing, dying, pruning back, adding new connections, storing old and new information, and adapting to changes in its environment. The growth and health of the Human Brain Project has depended in considerable part on the Internet's ability to provide instant and reasonably effective (and cheap) communication among scientists.

Those readers familiar with the history of science, and for that matter with the history of Western civilization, may detect something familiar here. More than 375 years ago, in 1609, Galileo Galilei built his first telescopes. Over the next several years he used this relatively new technology to look at heavenly bodies: the moon, the sun, the planet Jupiter, the planet Saturn, the Milky Way. So did others, including Thomas Herriot and Johannes Fabricius. Galileo discovered mountain ranges and great basins on the moon and four moons circling Jupiter. He discovered the real nature of the Milky Way—that it is made up of millions of stars. He even spotted Saturn's rings but didn't understand what they were. Herriot drew the first modern maps of the moon. Fabricius, Galileo, and several others all discovered sunspots at about the same time. The early 1600s were a momentous time for Western civilization. Creative men and a new technology came together at the same time, and the result was a scientific revolution that ultimately shook the foundations of Christendom. Out of their discoveries, and the brilliant insights of people like Newton and Leibniz, came a new paradigm, a new "framework" within which people could understand the nature of the world in which they lived.

Several years ago, in an interview for a book on the immune system, biochemist and immunologist Leroy Hood said that he believed science was actually pushed forward into new realms by technological breakthroughs. At the time, he was referring to the new gene-sequencing machines that he had helped invent. The Human Genome Project, of which he was a major proponent, is proof that he was correct. New generations of gene-sequencing technology are revolutionizing our understanding of our genetic makeup. However, that technology would be useless without the creative insights of people like Hood himself and the many other researchers who are rapidly deciphering the encyclopedia of genetic instructions for the human species. Together the researchers and the technology will create a world that, for good or ill, will be very different from the one in which we live today.

In a somewhat similar fashion, the researchers of the Human Brain Project and the new brain-imaging technologies they are using are providing us with new insights into the nature and function of the brain. From this work will come new explanations for terrible diseases, new cures for tragic brain-related conditions, and a new understanding of how we learn, remember, forget, speak, move, feel, and see.

And also how we think. The world that will grow out of these discoveries will be different from the one in which we live. How it will differ, we do not yet know. We have only the evidence of history, and of Galileo and his "optical tube," to tell us that it will likely be very different. The Decade of the Brain is just the beginning of what could easily turn out to be the Century of the Brain.

WHAT, THEN, is the real importance of the Decade of the Brain? Not gobs of new research money, certainly. Earlier we compared the Human Brain Project with the Internet. It is worth remembering that what the Internet is all about, in essence, is information and communication. And that may be what the Decade of the Brain is really about. In an interview for this book, Marcus Raichle, a pioneer in the use of positron-emission tomography (PET) for probing the workings of the living brain, said:

> I think people would hope that it would bring more resources to research. But the first thing that you have to do is to introduce the public, the people that pay these bills and who are concerned with these diseases, to what we are doing. And to the excitement

and the promise of this. For those of us who are caught up in it, it's every bit as exciting as sequencing the human genome, or figuring out what our origins were, or what the universe is all about. [The brain is] kind of like the universe within. It's really one of the last great scientific frontiers.

And you can relate to this at all sorts of levels. When somebody talks about some protein inserted in some calcium channel in a neuron somewhere, or about some piece of a genome, it's a little hard for the public to grasp what we are talking about. But when you talk about changes in the brain that are related to my feeling anxious, or changes in the brain that are related to my speaking or my seeing, it's not too hard to get a sense of that.

My feeling is that, if the Decade of the Brain establishes a better line of communication with the public who ultimately have to support this work, then we will have achieved a lot.

Back in 1609, Galileo had not the faintest idea that he was straddling a fault line. On one side, slipping away, was an old worldview. Under his other foot was a new world being born. Pressured and hounded by a church that let fear outweigh love and courage, Galileo tried to stand on both sides at once and couldn't quite do it. Who could?

Today, whether we know it or not, we also stand on a fault line. Purely by coincidence, it is running through a temporal territory called "the end of the millenium." That gives rise to a lot of outrageous pseudospiritual puffery. Nevertheless, the fault line is there. It is growing, wedged ever wider by some brilliant men and women using astonishing new machines to peer deep into the living workings of the greatest physical mystery of them all.

The mystery behind our eyes and between our ears.

The brain.

PART I

THE TERRITORY
AND THE MAPS

. . . my physicians by their love are grown
Cosmographers, and I their map, who lie
Flat on this bed . . . .
—JOHN DONNE, "Hymn to God, My God, in My Sickness"

CHAPTER 1

THE DECADE OF THE BRAIN

THANKSGIVING DAY, 1981, did not start out well for my youngest brother, Edward. For much of the previous week he'd been having terrible headaches. The pain at times had been so blinding that Ed could barely sit up. Eating had become out of the question; he would only vomit what he tried to ingest. He had called in sick at the supermarket where he was in charge of the produce section. It was a good job; he was rapidly moving up in both salary and responsibility while still taking classes at the local community college. But he hadn't been to classes for several days, either. The pain was too intense.

Finally, a day or two before Thanksgiving, his roommate had driven him from the apartment they shared to our parents' home near Ventura, California. My mother at the time was a registered nurse, working at St. John's Regional Medical Center in nearby Oxnard. Ed figured that whatever was wrong, Mom could probably help him out.

That Thanksgiving Day, he never left his bedroom. The headaches were so severe that he could hardly get out of bed to go to the bathroom. My parents were now quite alarmed. Though my mother at times suffered from migraine headaches, it was clear to her that whatever problem Ed had, it wasn't migraine. She made a decision: "We're going to the emergency room. Now." It was a good call. Unbeknownst to any of them, Ed was dying.

They bundled my brother into their car and drove him to St. John's and the emergency room. It was there that events started to turn in Ed's favor. The key to that turnaround was a still relatively new piece of medical imaging technology called a CAT scanner. In some ways a radically

9

souped up X-ray machine, the CAT scanner (now called a CT scanner) can produce astonishingly detailed X-ray images of the interior of the human body. X rays are great at creating good pictures of hard body parts, such as bones and cartilege, but are notoriously bad at imaging soft tissues, such as muscles and organs.

However, even in 1981 a CAT scanner could turn out a pretty good image of a soft-tissue organ like the brain. This was especially true if a special kind of dye was injected into the fluid that surrounds the spinal cord. This cerebrospinal fluid actually comes from the brain, and so the dye quickly returns to the brain's cavities or ventricles.

That's what the doctors did with my brother. They gave him an injection, right into the spinal column, of a dye that would quickly infuse the brain and provide greater definition and detail in the CAT-scan X rays. That such injections can be quite painful didn't matter much at that point to Edward.

The CAT scans revealed what no one had ever suspected. One of the tiny channels that drains cerebrospinal fluid from a ventricle at the rear of Ed's brain had become blocked. The fluid, instead of draining normally into his spinal column, was backing up into his brain like a stopped-up bathroom sink. The water in such a sink, though, eventually overflows. Stopped-up cerebrospinal fluid has nowhere to go. Fluid pressure builds up in the brain. First come the headaches and excruciating pain. Then comes unconsciousness. Then coma. Then death.

Drainpipes can get blocked by a buildup of hair, a toothpaste-tube top, or a piece of a child's toy. Ventricles get blocked by tissue. In Ed's brain a small tumor had been slowly growing, probably since he was an infant. Slowly, it grew, year after year, a tiny mass of tissue gradually expanding like a slow-motion explosion at the back of his head. It was not malignant, not cancerous; just tissue, possibly a small mass of neuroglia, a class of cells in the brain that provide neurons with insulation and structural support. It grew, in the wrong place and continuously. Now, after more than twenty years, it was killing my brother.

The CAT scans showed precisely where in the brain the blocking mass lay. That Thanksgiving night, Edward went under the surgeon's knife. The blockage could not be completely removed without causing even greater damage to his brain tissue in the area. So in order to open the ventricle and drain the fluid, the surgeon inserted a shunt.

The shunt is a thin piece of Teflon tubing. Teflon turns out to be good for more than nonstick kitchen pans. The immune system does not treat it as an "alien invader" of the body. And, of course, other body tissues are no more likely to stick to a piece of Teflon tube and pull it loose from its location than scrambled eggs will stick to the bottom of a Teflon-coated frying pan.

One end of the Teflon tube was inserted into the blocked ventricle in Ed's brain. The surgeon then threaded the tube down the right side of his throat, just underneath the skin, and into his chest cavity. Cerebrospinal fluid is quite harmless to organs in other parts of the body. Now the fluid in that particular ventricle would forevermore drain into Ed's chest and be naturally absorbed by the muscles and other tissues. The cerebrospinal fluid that built up in his other ventricles would continue to drain normally into his spine.

It took Ed several months to physically recover from the operation. He never resumed working at the supermarket, but he did finish community college. The psychological effects were longer term. He spent several years knocking about from job to job, looking for something to do that he could turn into a career. He's now in his mid-thirties and still doesn't have a "career." But he does have a job that pays well and that he greatly enjoys.

Other aspects of his life, those that really count, have improved. He is married to a woman named Marla, whom he deeply loves and who loves him. They have a young son, Tyler. They no longer live in Los Angeles, a city they came to deeply dislike, but in the mile-high, bustling city of Colorado Springs. The air's cleaner than in Los Angeles, the people are nicer, the skiing is much better, and it's a town in which my brother feels comfortable raising a family.

Many years have passed since that terrifying 1981 Thanksgiving. They are years my brother would never had had were it not for the new technologies of medical imaging that are revolutionizing the way we see and understand the human brain.

THE HUMAN BRAIN PROJECT

More than a decade after my brother's dance with death, it is a sunny autumn day in the City by the Bay. A carpet of ocean fog is slowly creeping over the tops of the ridges to the southwest, where the huge radio-television broadcast Sutro Tower stands guard. I drive up and down hilly streets, past neighborhood grocery stores and bay-windowed apartment buildings. Eventually, after a few wrong turns and frantic backtracks, I find what I seek: the University of California at San Francisco (UCSF) School of Medicine. After another several minutes spent reading a faxed map and locating a parking garage, I finally found the right building, the right office, and met the right man.

Joseph Martin is a distinguished-looking fellow in his late fifties. With his good looks, silvery hair, and white lab coat, he appears the perfect model for an archetypal movie scientist. Martin is a neurologist, someone who studies the working of the human nervous system. He has long been interested in studying inherited neurological disorders. That research led to a breakthrough in identifying a genetic "marker," or signpost, near the gene that probably causes many cases of Huntington's disease. His distinguished career in medical research eventually led him into administration; he is currently chancellor of UCSF.

In 1989, the same year he was appointed dean of UCSF's School of Medicine, he became involved with a government committee that eventually gave birth to the Human Brain Project. On that warm October late afternoon in San Francisco, we sat in Martin's UCSF offices on Parnassus Avenue, and he recalled the genesis of the Human Brain Project.

"Dr. Lou Judd, who was then the director of the National Institutes for Mental Health, approached me about a volunteer position he wanted me to take," he recalled. "Judd wanted to know if I would be willing to chair a panel of neuroscientists and clinical scientists from areas like psychiatry and neurology. They would study the issue of how to address the extraordinary complexity of neuroscience information. In particular, the committee would study how computer technology, and the computer's incredible capacity for data storage and analysis, could be helpful in taking this information and putting together the graphics of the brain."

Neuroscientists and anatomists know the brain as the three-dimensional organ it is. However, most of the rest of us—including most other scientists—see the brain only in pictures: in books or magazine articles or on TV. Even the amazing computer simulations now available to video producers end up being painted onto a two-dimensional television screen. "But we really have to think about the brain's functions in relation to its structure," Martin emphasized, "which has three-dimensional connectivity. Computer technology is very quickly expanding in that way. So it's now possible for one to use that new technology to both see the brain graphically and think about how to synthesize all this information into that three-dimensional representation."

The committee Judd wooed Martin into joining had the jaw-breaking name the National Neurocircuitry Data Base Committee. Martin, in fact, ended up chairing the committee. It carried on its work from 1989 through 1991, when it issued its final report. Said Martin, "I think the interesting thing about it was that we brought together people from very different worlds. For example, we had people from the computer fields who knew nothing about neuroscience. They knew how to program computers to do the things that we were interested in. And we had neuroscientists who might use Macs or word processors or who might do a little bit of graphics in relation to their own work but who didn't really know anything about big computer usage or networking or the Internet, and all that. Getting those two groups together and then having each educate the other about their fields so we could come up with some ideas on what direction to take was what the committee thought we could achieve pretty well."

"Pretty well" is a bit of an understatement. The committee's report actually became a bible of information and recommendations for integrating the vast amount of information about the human brain already flowing out of labs around the world. Researchers and administrators in government agencies, academic institutions, and even corporate medical labs took it to heart. The report written by Martin and his committee quickly led to funding from the National Institutes of Health (NIH) through its various agencies for a new effort to map the human brain. It is this effort that has come to be known as the Human Brain Project.

An important symbolic (if not financial) impetus to the Human Brain Project was the joint congressional declaration of "the Decade of the Brain." On June 29, 1989, the House of Representatives passed House Joint Resolution (HJR) 174. The Senate followed suit on July 13. HJR 174 was then signed by President George Bush and became Public Law 101-58. In HJR 174 the Senate and House resolved that "the decade beginning January 1, 1990, hereby [be] designated 'Decade of the Brain'." The resolution also "authorized and requested" that the president "issue a proclamation calling upon all public officials and the people of the United States to observe such decade with appropriate programs and activities."

The declaration of the 1990s as the Decade of the Brain focused the nation's attention on the importance of brain research and on the opportunities for advancing our knowledge of this most complex of human organs. The years that have followed HJR 174 have seen brain researchers the world over begin to make the Decade of the Brain more than just a noble-sounding political platitude. With not much additional governmental funding but an enormous amount of creativity, ingenuity, and increasingly sophisticated technological tools, researchers are fashioning the ad hoc Human Brain Project into a powerful engine of discovery and, eventually, healing. The marvelously designed organ within our skulls that allows us to learn, remember, plan, decide, and communicate, that governs our bodies and perhaps even creates our minds, is beginning to yield its secrets.

The first NIH grants for the Human Brain Project were funded in October 1992, and the agency has continued to support the effort. Most of the leadership for the Human Brain Project has come from the National Institute of Mental Health (NIMH), said Martin. Funding for the project has been divided among fifty different agencies and has reached a level of about $15 million a year. This may seem like a huge amount, but it is actually only about one-tenth of the funds currently being pumped into the much better known Human Genome Project. Despite that, Martin feels that the brain-mapping project is off to a good start. He is excited about the progress that is being made and expects many more advances in the years to come.

According to Martin, three consortia have been put together to handle the NIH's brain-mapping grants. "The idea is to bring together people who are working in an area of neuroscience or computer science and have them communicate with each other through the Internet and other mechanisms," he explained. "That way, one isn't limited to one's own institution."

One consortium is led by Floyd Bloom, a pioneer in the early groundbreaking studies of the brain chemicals known as endorphins. He also became deeply involved in the rise of the Human Genome Project and its efforts to map the human genetic code and is the current editor of the prestigious journal *Science*. According to Martin, Bloom's brain-mapping consortium is trying to connect maps of human and rodent brains with information on brain chemicals and the connections between brain cells (or neurons). "This is a kind of descriptive project that will allow people to quickly get into what's already known," Martin explained. "It will be important for educational purposes, and eventually it will help to facilitate research."

A second consortium, led by Peter Fox, is working on PET (positron-emission tomography) scanning and MRI (magnetic resonance imaging). Like Bloom, Fox is also the editor of an influential medical journal, one that focuses on brain imaging. As we'll see in more detail later on, PET and MRI are two medical imaging technologies that are revolutionizing the study of the human brain. The third consortium is doing work that Martin finds particularly interesting. This group is based at the California Institute of Technology, or Cal Tech, in Pasadena, California, and is headed by David Brower. According to Martin, Brower's consortium is exploring some new and experimental way to map the brain.

BRAIN AND GENOME

It is perhaps inevitable that people will make comparisons between the Human Brain Project and the Human Genome Project. One obvious parallel is the relationship between biology and computer science. Both the Human Genome Project and the new brain-mapping effort require getting biology people together with computer people. The biologists and geneticists are the "wet science" people. They work in messy little laboratories where until recently they couldn't imagine having a computer. Everyone knows that computers and liquids don't mix. Try spilling coffee on your keyboard, for example. Then there are the circuits people, men and women who spend all their time immersed in the virtual reality of electrons, chips, and supercomputers. The first major hurdle for the Human Genome Project, back in 1989 and 1990, was getting these two groups together and creating a common language. The successful leaping of the hurdle has been directly responsible for the accelerating pace of the project.

Martin agreed that clear parallels exist between the Human Genome Project and the Human Brain Project. However, he added, one very important difference also exists between the two. "Much of the initial information about the human genome is linear," he said. "You have three billion base pairs of DNA in the human genetic code," and we essentially map the code by going from base-pair number one to 3 billion. "It's a linear problem. But the brain," he continued with a smile and a rising voice, "is ten orders of magnitude more complex than the human genetic code. You've got its structure, its functions, its relationships, and its three-dimensional aspects. And then there's the fact that probably half of the hundred thousand human genes that are going to be discovered in the human genome deal with the brain in determining its proteins. So one has not only to consider the brain as a nonlinear system, for it is three-dimensional and has connectivity at submicroscopic, microscopic, and gross levels. You also have all the genes that are expressed underneath all of that. The genes are what make it possible for the brain to develop, to make its connections, to form its neurotransmitters, such as endorphins and other brain chemicals, so you'll end up with a structure that can actually work.

"So it's just mind-boggling to think about how much more complex the brain is than the human genome."

BASIC RESEARCH AND COGNITIVE SCIENCE

Basic neuroscience explores the brain and nervous system to discover the fundamental ways in which neurons work, how the nervous system develops, and how the brain has evolved adaptations for appropriate behavior in particular environments. The discoveries are the building blocks needed to answer questions about the brain, behavior, intelligence, and disease. The human brain is a vastly complex organ and until recently has been largely inaccessible to detailed research. The problem is not so much that it lies sheltered within its cage of bone. Rather, almost any attempt at physically probing a living human brain runs the serious risk of causing severe—even fatal—damage to the patient. For this reason, organizations like the National Science Foundation (NSF) have usually supported research on comparatively simple biological systems and on new ways of extracting information from human behavior. A simple system can be nothing more than a few brain cells growing in a petri dish in a totally controlled setting. It can be the brain of an invertebrate,° like an insect with a few hundred cells, or subsystems in the brains of vertebrates. Brain research on vertebrate biological systems range from evolutionarily ancient species, such as the lamprey, all the way to studies of human brains. Until recently, most basic biological research on human brains has been on a dissecting table—what researchers call in vitro (Latin for "on glass"). Since the early 1980s, however, researchers have begun doing basic research on living human brains with high-tech imaging technology.

° Invertebrates are animals that do not have backbones, such as insects, jellyfishes, flatworms, and mollusks. Vertebrates are animals that do have backbones.

The studies of human behavior supported by the NSF and other organizations have usually included research in human perception, in various areas of linguistics (the science of language), in developmental and social psychology, and in physical and cultural anthropology. In recent years another discipline has been added: the growing area of cognitive science. Cognitive science is an interdisciplinary activity that focuses on understanding "intelligent systems," whether biological or artificial.

Of course, no artificial-intelligence systems exist—yet. But many people besides science fiction writers are convinced that such entities will someday exist. If and when they do, their presence among us will only serve to throw into greater relief those questions that have been puzzling humans for as long as they have been human:

- What is the nature of thought?
- What is consciousness?
- What is "mind?"
- How do we learn and use language?
- How do we understand each other?
- How do we even recognize one another, by being able to identify shapes and faces?

Researchers in anthropology, computer science, linguistics, neurobiology, philosophy, psychology, and sociology have for years been looking for answers to these questions, but always from their own shuttered points of view. Cognitive science has developed from the interaction among and between people working in these oft-seeming different fields. Their common goal, and the goal of cognitive science, is twofold. The first is to understand the human mind using each discipline's own tools and methods. The second is to integrate this knowledge into an overarching theory of the brain and its thought processes.

The rise of the computer as an enormous agent of change in our society has only served to spur cognitive scientists to new heights of creativity.

THE COMPUTER AND COGNITIVE SCIENCE

A technological advance wrought in the fires of World War II provided the impetus for not only a whole new set of cognitive questions but for some rather intriguing new spins on the perennial ones. That breakthrough was the development of the first electronic computer. Howard Aiken, a mathematician at Harvard University, spearheaded the development of the Mark I, a computer that used more than three-thousand electromechanical relays as on-off switches. The Mark I was finished in 1944 and was used by the U.S. Navy to create ballistics tables for accurate artillery.

The Mark I used mechanical relays powered by electricity. The first fully electronic computer used vacuum tubes as on-off switches. It had been in use a full year before Mark I came on-line, but it would be decades before anyone other than a small group of initiates would know about it. Called Colossus, it was invented by the English mathematician Alan M. Turing and was used by British cryptographers to break secret German military codes.

The first modern general-purpose electronic computer was ENIAC, or electronic numerical integrator and calculator. Designed by American engineers John Mauchly and J. Presper Eckert, ENIAC was plugged in at the University of Pennsylvania in 1946. The thirty-ton machine contained 17,468 vacuum tubes linked by five hundred miles of wiring. ENIAC performed one hundred thousand operations per second.

Early electronic computers like ENIAC and UNIVAC were gargantuan in size, but later generations of so-called mainframe computers fit comfortably in single, large air-conditioned rooms. The invention of the transistor in 1948 made this early "miniaturization" possible. Unlike vacuum tubes, transistors generated little heat and functioned perfectly as switches or amplifiers. In 1958 American engineer Jack Kilby designed the first true integrated circuit. It included transistors, resistors, and capacitors—the major components of electronic circuitry. Thirteen years later, Marcian E. Hoff created the microprocessor, the Intel 4004, essentially an entire computer on one tiny silicon chip.

The 1950s saw large mainframe computers beginning to be used as tools for research. Meanwhile, cognitive science itself was getting its start as an integrated field of with the publication of several important papers on categorization, memory, and linguistic theory.

By the mid-1970s, the cost of the electronic components of a computer had dropped so radically that "ordinary people" could begin playing the game that large corporations like IBM had until then kept to themselves. In the 1960s and 1970s computer hobbyists began building simple but impressive computers that fit on the top of a table. The first affordable desktop computer designed specifically for personal use appeared in 1974: the Altair 8800. Three years later, the Tandy

Corporation became the first major electronics firm to produce a personal computer. They added a keyboard and monitor to their computer (the Altair 8800 had neither) as well as a way of storing computer instructions (today called programs or software) on a cassette recorder.

A year later, the computer revolution began in earnest. Budding businessman Steven Jobs and his engineer pal Stephen Wozniak had literally been building desktop computers they called the Apple I in their garage. Now they formed their own company, Apple Computers, and began producing a desktop computer far superior to Tandy's offering. Three years later, IBM finally produced its personal computer (PC). The price of personal computers fell drastically as hundreds of companies old and new quickly began producing copies, or "clones," of the IBM-PC. Today's personal computer is two hundred times faster than ENIAC, three thousand times lighter, and several million dollars cheaper. Laptop and palmtop computers are now commonplace.

At nearly the same time the two Steves were revolutionizing the hardware end of computers, two other young Turks were revamping the software side. Paul Allen and Bill Gates III had started a small company called Microsoft Corporation. IBM, huge in both size and overconfidence, had gambled that the personal-computer fad would fade. Instead, the rules of the game they had run for years suddenly changed on them. Now they were desperate to get back on the field with their IBM-PC. They contracted with Allen and Gates to produce the operating system for their new desktop machine. The operating system, or OS, is the set of instructions that makes it possible for a computer to compute and run other computer programs. The Microsoft Operating System, or MS-DOS, was what they created. IBM decided to make its computer and operating system an "open system" so that others could easily create computer programs that would run on their computers. (Apple, by contrast, played its hardware and operating system cards close to the vest with a "closed system.") This decision eventually created the PC clone industry. It also made Gates and Allen multimillionaires, as MS-DOS became the operating system of choice on untold millions of PCs and PC clones. Soon others jumped into the software fray, creating a myriad of clever, exciting, powerful, and useful programs to run on desktop computers. Many of them went broke; many became millionaires, too. It eventually became clear that the computer revolution was not just a matter of revolutionary machines but also of revolutionary new ways to tell those machines what to do and how to do it.

And therein lies the connection between the modern electronic computer revolution and cognitive science. Knowing what they now know about the immense physical complexity of the human brain, researchers are asking questions about the physiological basis of thought and the human mind. How do the billions of highly interconnected cells that form our brains give rise to the complex set of cognitive abilities demonstrated by human thought? Can computers help us better understand human thought and the human mind? Conversely, how can our increasing knowledge of human thinking improve the nature and functioning of electronic computers? And the big question: Will computers ever be able to "think" or "reason" like humans? Will computers ever become conscious? Will our silicon-chip creations develop minds of their own?

IN 1984, Dr. Richard Restak published *The Brain*, a thoroughly engaging and perceptive look at the then-current status of brain research. More than a decade has passed since then, and much has happened. In particular, three significant technological developments have emerged that are making possible the novel findings of present research on the human brain and nervous system. First, brain researchers are now making use of the tools of molecular genetics. They use DNA clones and probes to study the brain at the molecular level, examine how different genes code for the creation (or "expression," as molecular biologists say) of proteins in the brain, and study examples of both normal and abnormal neural structure and function.

Second, an explosion of new anatomic techniques enables neuroscientists to trace pathways and to identify particular cell types. These include new kinds of stains and dyes for studying individual cells and doing real-time monitoring of large groups of brain cells, new techniques for identifying and labeling specific types or classes of cells, and new kinds of microscopes for studying living tissue.

Finally, computers are now to be found in virtually every laboratory. This allows researchers to study events happening in the brain in extraordinarily tiny time slices. They can now carry out real-time analysis of their data. And, of course, today's midrange and desktop computers give researchers tremendous data-capture and storage capabilities. Some researchers are even using supercomputers to develop new theories about much more complex systems of model neurons than was ever before possible.

But the most exciting development is one that is the result of the *ménage à trois* of hardware, software, and "wetware." Of computers, computer programs, and neurobiology. Neuroscientists are now using noninvasive imaging technologies to scan the activity of living human brains. PET, MRI, and other physical imaging methods are now making possible astonishing new discoveries about the brain. Advances in brain-imaging techniques, computer modeling, and neurophysiology have increased our understanding of how the brain works, second by second. For the first time, cognitive scientists have the technological tools needed to scientifically answer some of those fundamental philosophical questions about perception, memory, learning, language, and the nature of consciousness itself.

It is in this arena that the two major foci of basic brain research—the study of biological systems and of human behavior—meet. Government research agencies, universities, and private companies around the globe are devoting enormous efforts to basic laboratory experiments meant to answer key questions:

- How does the brain produce behavior?
- How does the human brain use the input from our senses to control bodily movement?
- What are the interactions between the nervous system and the endocrine system, the set of glands that produces chemicals called hormones?
- What can the study of behavior in many animal species tell us about the human brain and human behavior?

Even at the current levels of financial support, researchers are using their fantastic new tools to make astonishing and provocative break-throughs. The Decade of the Brain promises to produce results that will make it possible for us to explain ourselves to ourselves and to make new breakthroughs in medicine, substance abuse, and yes, perhaps even the creation of artificial intelligence.

Those results are already beginning to appear.

CHAPTER 2

THE BRAIN FROM BOTTOM TO TOP

MOST OF US, without having any knowledge of human physiology, can enjoy watching a dance troupe perform. We can dance ourselves—swing or slam, frug or line, boogie-woogie or square—with no intellectual understanding of the science of movement. We can walk; we can dance. However, if we want to dance professionally, we should learn a little kinesiology, the science of how the body moves. A little knowledge of how the body works, or of the science of movement, can also increase the layperson's appreciation of dance as an art form. The same holds true of the mind and brain.

THE BUILDING BLOCKS OF THE BRAIN

Like every other organ or tissue in the body, the human brain is composed of cells. A cell is the smallest unit of living matter that can exist by itself. Some living creatures are single-celled. The amoeba is a good example. Others, including humans, are composed of many trillions of cells.

Most cells are so tiny, they cannot be seen with the unaided eye. Their size is usually measured in microns; 1 micron is about .000039 inch. The average cell in the human body is about 10 microns in diameter.

All cells consist of a watery substance called protoplasm and have three major structures: the cell membrane, the cytoplasm, and the nucleus. The membrane is the cell's complex and semipermeable "skin." Most of the cell's chemical activity is carried out in the cytoplasm, the protoplasm within the membrane. The nucleus, in turn, is walled off from the cytoplasm by its own membrane and is the cell's control center. Here is found the material of the cell's genetic code, the DNA that comprises genes and chromosomes.

The brain consists primarily of two types of cells. Neurons are the information-carrying cells of the brain. Their electrochemical activity is really what the brain is all about. All available evidence to date reveals that our memories, feelings, impulses, and even thoughts are the product of the actions of neurons. The brain contains about 100 billion neurons—as many neurons in the brain as there are stars in the Milky Way galaxy.

The other main type of brain cell is the glial cell, also known as glia. Glia fit into the spaces between neurons. They are the "glue" that holds the neurons together in a myriad of complex structures. The brain contains ten to a hundred times as many neuroglia as neurons.

Neurons in the central nervous system ordinarily cannot reproduce themselves. Damaged neurons can usually begin again and create new networks in the brain. But actual reproduction of new brain cells is nearly always impossible. If the nerve tissue of the brain or spinal cord is severely injured, the damage is permanent. Messages from other neurons cannot travel past the point of injury, which is why such injuries usually result in permanent paralysis or even death. In recent years,

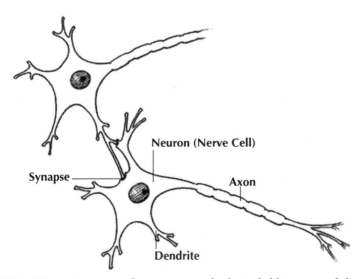

FIG. 2.1. Two major parts of a neuron are the branch-like axon and dendrites. The tiny gap between the end of one neuron's axon and another neuron is called the synapse. It is here that chemicals transfer information from one neuron to the next.

though, some research and experimental work with nerve-growth factors has begun to offer hope for some limited regeneration of actual nerve cells in the brain and spinal cord.

THE SYNAPTIC SYMPHONY

Neurons are connected to one another through circuits called synapses. But unlike the tiny pathways in your computer that connect to one another to make an electrical circuit, synapses never quite touch one another. The signal from one neuron to the next must jump the gap between them. It does so not with a microscopic bolt of electricity but by means of a wave of chemicals.

Imagine that the neuron is a small bottle suspended in water. The bottle is also filled with water, but under pressure, and for the sake of our scenario, the water in the bottle is a bright blue. The bottle's walls are also quite thin. In some places, such as the top of the bottle's neck, the walls are downright fragile. As long as the walls hold, the pressurized water will stay inside the bottle. Now suppose someone suddenly shakes the bottle—hard. The fragile skin at the neck of the bottle fractures. The blue water in the bottle spurts out of the opening. Now, it just so happens that another similar bottle is suspended very close to the first one. The blue water pouring out of the tiny fracture in the first bottle crosses the tiny space between the two and hits the wall of the second bottle. The impact causes the water in the second bottle to pulse back and forth. The sudden buildup of pressure is just enough to fracture a tiny part of the second bottle's wall, and the process continues.

Instead of water and pressure, substitute electrical charges and voltages and you will have an idea of how neurons send signals to one another across the synaptic gaps. Of course, it's considerably more complicated than this simple analogy. One complication is worth mentioning: neurotransmitters.

A neurotransmitter is simply a chemical released by one neuron into the gap between it and another neuron. Some of the neurotransmitter molecules interact with tiny regions, or "receptors," on the skin of the neighboring neuron. The neurotransmitters are like keys, and the receptor molecules are the locks into which they fit. The neurotransmitter "unlocks" the receptor. If enough locks get opened, the neuron may fire off its own signal, continuing the chain. Some neurotransmitters, however, *prevent* neurons from firing. One can begin to glimpse how complex these interactions among brain cells can get.

THE NERVOUS SYSTEM

The human brain is the part of the central nervous system inside the skull. It looks a little like a mushroom or a broccoli floret atop its stalk. The rest of the central nervous system is the thin rope of nerve tissue called the spinal cord, which runs down from the base of the brain through the spine.

From the spinal cord branch the nerves that make up the peripheral nervous system. Thirty-one different nerve fibers branch out from the front, or ventral side, of the spinal cord (the side that faces your stomach and lungs), like off-ramps, on-ramps, and smaller roads from a busy superhighway, and reach into the rest of the body. These motor nerves carry instructions from the brain to the body's skin, muscles, and organs. Another thirty-one nerve fibers enter the rear, or *dorsal* side, of the spinal column (the side facing your back). These sensory fibers carry information from the body's internal and external sensory detectors, sending it up the spinal cord and into the brain. Another thirteen pairs of nerve fibers, called the cranial nerves, originate in the head. The brain sends and receives signals through the peripheral nervous system. Oxygen and food travel into the brain through an intricate network of arteries carrying blood.

The brain itself is a grayish-pink ball of tissue with the consistency of cooked oatmeal. Its surface is marked by numerous fissures and ridges that give it a striking wrinkled appearance. Those wrinkles, by the way, enormously increase its actual surface area. Only about a third of the brain's surface area is visible. If an adult brain could be "unfolded" so that its ridges and grooves were completely flattened out, its total surface area would be nearly 2,100 square centimeters, about 324 square inches. That's more than one and a half times the area of a twenty-inch diagonal television screen and twelve times the area of a page of a standard-sized paperback book. The typical adult human brain has a volume of 1,400 cubic centimeters (around 85 cubic inches), about that of three pints of milk.

THE THREEFOLD BRAIN

The brain has three main parts: the forebrain, the midbrain, and the hindbrain. The human forebrain distinguishes it from all other creatures

on the planet. This is particularly true of the part of the forebrain called
the cerebrum. In fish, the cerebrum is nothing more than a tiny swelling
at the front of the brain that processes olfactory information. Fish smell
with their forebrains. And for fish smell is very important, since chemicals diffuse very quickly through water. In humans, though, the cerebrum is the top part of the brain. A deep crevice divides the cerebrum
into two distinct halves, called the left and right cerebral hemispheres.
Each hemisphere controls the movement and sensory functions of the
opposite side of the body. Thus, the left hemisphere controls the right
arm, leg, toes, and fingers as well as sensory input from the right ear and
the skin on the right side of our bodies. The right hemisphere controls
the left arm, leg, toes, and so on.

A layer of gray matter, called the cortex, covers the outer part of
the cerebrum. Underneath the gray matter of the cortex is a layer of
cells called white matter. The cortex itself is wrinkled with ridges and
grooves.

Brain scientists traditionally divide the cerebrum's two hemispheres
into four separate lobes (which are often also called cortexes). They are
the frontal lobe, at the front of the brain; the parietal lobe, which runs
along the top of the brain; the occipital lobe, at the back of the brain;
and the left and right temporal lobes, lying just below the frontal and
parietal lobes, at about the location of the ears (Fig. 2.2).

Each of the four lobes appears to have specific functions that the
others do not. Also, considerable evidence exists that each of the two
cerebral hemispheres handles certain kinds of processes that the other
does not. This specialization is called brain lateralization. The popular
but erroneous idea that we each have "two brains" is based on the legitimate existence of brain lateralization. The "left brain–right brain" idea
has spawned a small but highly profitable industry of self-help books,
workshops, psychotherapeutic disciplines, art classes, and New Age reli-
gious practices. In fact, we each have one brain with two cerebral hemispheres. The hemispheres do have lateralized functions. But they also
communicate with one another constantly through a thick band of nerve
tissue called the corpus callosum. The remarkable advances in brain
imaging have revealed new details about brain lateralization. These
findings simply don't support the left brain–right brain idea, but they
have given us new insights into how the brain *really* functions, including
the role of lateralization in language, body movement, and even some
mental illnesses.

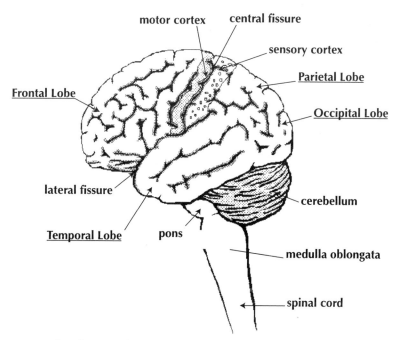

FIG. 2.2.   This drawing shows the major divisions and surface features of the human brain. This view has the front of the brain facing left and thus the left hemisphere facing the viewer.

Deep in the forebrain are several other important regions. One is the limbic system, which might be thought of as "Emotion Central" for the human brain. The basal ganglia are another set of important brain structures in the cerebrum. The basal ganglia help control our physical movement. The hypothalamus regulates body temperature, hunger, thirst, and breathing rate. It influences blood pressure and plays a crucial role during puberty in the development of secondary sexual characteristics. The pituitary gland is the source of numerous hormones that act as master controllers of other glands in the body. The pituitary, in turn, is controlled by chemical triggers released by the hypothalamus.

The other two main anatomic parts of the brain are the midbrain and the hindbrain. The midbrain is an inch-long band of nerve fibers lying at the very base of the brain, underneath the forebrain. An area of the midbrain called the substantia nigra (in Latin, "black stuff") helps coordinate movement and muscle tone. Other parts of the midbrain receive sensory information from the eyes and ears as well as input from the cerebrum above. The midbrain helps control eye movement and some muscular reflexes. The ability of the eye's pupil to adjust to different light levels, for example, is controlled by the midbrain.

The hindbrain has several distinctive structures. The cerebellum (the name literally means "little cerebrum") accounts for one-eighth of the brain's total mass. It looks a bit like a cabbage and lies below the occipital lobe and above the brain stem. Like the cerebrum, it is divided into two hemispheres. The cerebellum helps control our body's position and muscular coordination. It also plays a major role in some emotions, especially anger and pleasure.

The pons is a band of nerve cells about an inch long, lying below the midbrain, which serves as the link between the midbrain and the cerebellum. The brain stem is the part of the hindbrain that lies below the cerebellum and connects the rest of the brain to the spinal cord. The medulla oblongata is the lowermost part of the brain stem. It includes regions that control reflexes, such as swallowing, heartbeat, blood pressure, breathing, and—interestingly enough—sneezing. It is also the way station for messages traveling to and from the body. At the very rear of the medulla is the reticular formation, a network of cells that spread throughout the brain stem. It controls or influences alertness, waking, sleeping, and various automatic reflexes.

MORE BRAIN FACTS

The brain of a newborn baby weighs less than half a kilogram (a bit over a pound), but it grows quickly. This growth is not the result of the creation of additional neurons or brain cells. We are each born with nearly all the brain cells we'll ever possess. What *do* grow, however, are the neurons already present. The connections between neurons and among different groups of neurons multiply at an astonishing rate. At the same time, connections between neurons and neuron clusters that the brain does not use end up atrophying. But the explosive growth of other interconnections and networks more than makes up for these losses in brain mass. By the time the child is six years old, the brain has already reached its final weight of about 1.4 kilograms (around 3 pounds). It is no coincidence that the fastest rate of learning and acquiring new behavior patterns takes place during the first six years of a person's life. For example, just consider language. The average human progresses from zero language skills at birth to expressing and understanding the meaning of individual words by the age of one year. By the time a child is four or five, he or she can speak and understand sentences and carry on simple but meaningful conversations with others. What's more, untold millions of children achieve this astonishing task twice over. They are raised in bilingual households and learn two languages more or less at the same time.

Our brains are the neurological rulers of our bodies, the "master control." The brain receives information about the world beyond our bodies through senses such as sight and hearing. The brain also continuously acquires information about the body's condition from various internal sensors. It constantly knows the position and rate of movement of our arm and hand as we lift a cup of coffee to our mouths; how and by how much our torso and head twist as we turn to say hello to someone; the temperature of the coffee in our mouths—ouch! too hot!—and the tenseness in our muscles as we recognize the person as an enemy.

The brain continuously analyzes all the data it receives, acts on it when necessary, and stores it as memories of various kinds. Certain clusters of memory-data (smell, taste, color, temperature) mean "coffee." Other memory data patterns equal a familiar face—our mother, our husband, a new adversary, an old friend whom we haven't seen in thirty years. Then there is thought, reasoning, imagination, fantasy. All, as far as we know, are generated by the brain. The mind, in other words, is probably just the brain at work.

All that work means the brain needs a lot of food. The human brain accounts for only about 2 percent of the body's total weight. But it uses up to 20 percent of the oxygen consumed by the entire body—and that's at rest. If the brain is deprived of oxygen for only a few minutes, serious damage can result. An intricate network of blood vessels supplies the brain the huge amounts of food and oxygen it needs to run at full capacity. Moreover, the brain's voracious need for oxygen and food is what makes today's amazing brain-imaging technologies possible. As we'll soon see, imaging devices like positron-emission tomography (PET) and magnetic resonance imaging (MRI) depend on the brain's massive use of oxygen and glucose, a form of sugar.

The result of billions of years of evolution, the human nervous system is designed to carry out two vital functions. It monitors and dynamically maintains the internal status of the body, and it provides the organism with information about the outside world. All these data travel to and from the brain through the nerves. If you've ever done any wiring in your house, you're probably familiar with "Romex." Romex is a thick electrical cable that is actually several smaller wires wrapped together. In somewhat the same way, a nerve is a bundle of thin extensions of nerve cells.

Nerves are one-way streets. Information coming from a temperature sensor in the skin of the hand, for example, travels to the brain through one nerve. If the brain interprets the data as "Too hot! Danger! Move!" its instructions to move must return to the hand through a separate nerve. Sensory (or efferent) nerves are the conduits for information traveling from the body's sense organs and other body receptors. They carry the information to the spinal cord and brain for processing. Motor (or afferent) nerves carry instructions for action from the brain, through the spinal cord, to the body's muscles and glands.

THE BRAIN AND THE COMPUTER

Many of us have the somewhat mistaken idea that the human brain is very much like a computer. The truth is, no computer of steel and silicon has ever worked like the "computer" between our ears. True, some similarities exist. In both the brain and a computer, electrical signals move along pathways we could call circuits. Both the brain and a computer store, process, and retrieve information from these circuits. But there the similarity ends. The computer on your desk at work or in the family room at home contains circuits made of silicon and metal. The brain creates its electrical signals using chemicals. The myriad elements of those circuits, the brain cells or neurons, are also tiny bags of membranes and chemicals. The different connections between and among brain cells are actually not really connections at all: they never quite touch one another. No desktop computer ever rewired itself on the fly. Human brains do it all the time. And a desktop computer's complexity and power fade to insignificance when compared to the human brain. Gigabyte hard disks, floppy disks, ROM memory, RAM memory, motherboards, modems—brush them all aside. The most powerful computers currently in existence, such as the Cray supercomputers or Thinking Machine, Inc.'s massively parallel computers, may equal the computing power of a grasshopper brain. The human brain is light-years beyond them in complexity and information-processing ability.

One stunning way to get a sense of the human brain's immense complexity is to examine the number and nature of the connections among its neurons. Neuroscientists call the connection between two neurons a synapse. It is roughly—*very* roughly—similar to the connections between electronic switches in a computer. These switches, which are built into the computer's microchips, must be either open or closed. That means they transmit information in binary form, as 0's or 1's. It's either on or off, yes or no. The synapses or connections among neurons in the human brain are immensely more complex than this, for they do not necessarily transmit data in pure binary form.

But let's suppose they do and start with a very simple "brain" having just two neurons and one binary-type connection between them. Such a brain can exist in only one of two possible informational states—no or yes. If this simple two-neuron brain had two synapses or connections between the neurons, it would have not two but four potential mental states: yes and no, yes and yes, no and yes, or no and no. What about three synapses connecting the two neurons? Now there are *eight* possible states for this simple brain: yes, yes, and yes; yes, yes, and no; yes, no, and no; yes, no, and yes; no, no, and no; no, no, and yes; no, yes, and no; or no, yes, and yes.

We can represent each set of these possible yes-no states in a simple mathematical fashion, as X^y (Fig. 2.1). The big number represents the possible states of the synapse. In this case it's 2, for yes or no, on or off. The superscript number, in turn, represents the actual number of synapses connecting the two neurons in our simple brain. So the total number of potential states of a two-neuron brain with one synapse is 2^1, or 2. The total number of potential states with two synapses is 2^2, or 4 (2 squared, or 2×2), and of three synapses is 2^3, or 8 (2 cubed, or $2 \times 2 \times 2$).

Now, though, the numbers start getting interesting. If our two-cell brain has four synapses, it can have sixteen mental states (2^4); five, 32 states (2^5). Ten synapses yield 1,024 possible yes-no states (2^{10}).

Neuroscientists estimate that the human brain contains about 100 billion neurons and that each of those neurons has an *average* of a thousand connections, or synapses, with other neurons. Many neurons, of course, have far fewer connections to other brain cells. Others, such as the neurons in the cerebellum, have a hundred thousand or more connections with other neurons. Overall, though, this adds up to about 100 *trillion* synapses, or interconnections, in the brain. Imagine, for a moment, a simple two-cell brain with 100 trillion connections between the two neurons. That's $2^{100,000,000,000,000}$ potential yes-no brain-state combinations. That's a number larger than the number of atoms in the universe.

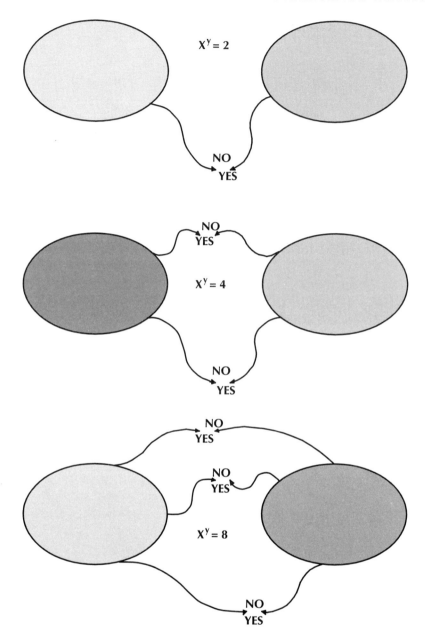

FIG. 2.3. How the number of possible connections in the brain rapidly increase.

But this is not a simple two-cell brain we're talking about. It's a human brain with 100 billion neurons sharing 100 trillion connections. Nor are these connections randomly distributed. The brain's neurons are arranged in an incredibly intricate structure of layers, columns, rows, ovoids, and fans. And each of these structures, in turn, contains other structures of neurons. To top it all off, the brain is nothing at all like a computer, using the simple binary language of zeros and ones, nor do neurons—as we'll soon discover—function like tiny transistors or microchips. It is not uncommon, for example, for the synapses from one neuron to physically influence the transmission state of a second neuron's connections to a *third* brain cell.

What's more, the human brain *learns*. Some sets of neuronal connections can be strengthened, while others are ignored or die off. Computer scientists have spent decades figuring out how to get computer circuits to mimic this process. Indeed, they call the kinds of circuits that learn from experience *neural* networks. The real neural networks are the ones constantly interacting within the 1.4 kilos of oatmeallike tissue between your ears. They are the most recent products of billions of years of evolution.

And conjured up from this electrochemical swirl of signals locked inside our skulls, like a spell cast by a sorcerer, is the mystery we call the mind.

CHAPTER 3

THE MAPPING MACHINES

OVER THE LAST TEN YEARS or so a dedicated cadre of men and women around the world have begun using fantastic new machines to peer deep into recesses of the human brain. Slowly but surely, they are uncovering the answers to some of the greatest mysteries of life:

- How do we perceive the reality outside our skins?
- How does the brain control our body's movements?
- Where does language come from, and how does the brain store words and phrases?
- What is memory? How do we learn?
- Why do some things go terribly wrong within the brain, resulting in mental illnesses, such as schizophrenia and depression, and physical ailments like Alzheimer's disease?
- What is the nature of human consciousness and self-awareness?
- And, perhaps most importantly, what is the mind itself, and what, if anything, is its connection to the spongy ball of tissue and fluid that lies caged behind our faces?

MAKING MAPS OF THE BRAIN

Ever since the Renaissance, when doctors and others began conducting (at first, illegal) autopsies on the bodies of dead criminals, scientists have known what the brain looks like. Over the years they built up a considerable body of knowledge about the physical structure of the brain. The invention of the microscope and its use in medicine vastly increased our understanding of the brain's physical makeup. At the beginning of the twentieth-century, Golgi and Ramón y Cajal developed new techniques for staining nerve cells and discovered the synaptic nature of information transmission in the brain and nervous system.

However, many of the methods used to map the human brain were, until very recently, only applicable to *dead* human brains. Brains would be removed from cadavers and sliced, diced, sampled, poked, and puréed in efforts to determine their fine structure. Scientists learned an enormous amount about the brain from these kinds of studies, but the information was "static" and provided little knowledge about the dynamic workings of living human brains.

Other researchers, meanwhile, were indeed gaining new insights into the workings of the living brain, but in a somewhat backward manner. These scientists studied people who had suffered cerebral "accidents": strokes, for example, or severe brain injuries from car crashes or other traumas. Some people who survived these experiences would turn out to have lost certain brain functions. A patient might be able to write fluently but be unable to speak a word. Another person might be able to identify a hammer but not her husband. Still another patient might have lost all ability to identify colors—including even the *concept* of "color." These oftentimes bizarre side effects of strokes and other brain injuries researchers dubbed "natural experiments." By identifying the areas of the brain that were injured or destroyed by a cerebral accident, scientists could connect them to the kinds of brain processes the person had lost. Slowly they began to build maps of the brain that connected function with structure.

However, these two main methods of brain mapping—studying "natural experiments" in living people and examining the detailed structure in autopsied brains—remained more or less unconnected to one another. Beginning in the early 1970s, though, a series of technological breakthroughs began that would lead to the creation of machines and techniques that would bridge this gap. This was the development of noninvasive methods of probing the living brain. The best known of these new tools are computerized tomographic imaging (CT), positron-emission tomography (PET), and magnetic resonance imaging (MRI). An older imaging tool, still used with considerable frequency and effectiveness, is electroencephalography (EEG). These exciting new technologies have all been built on the work of physicists, doctors, mathematicians, and engineers who lived in the eighteenth and nineteenth centuries. In fact, the first form of noninvasive medical imaging was developed more than a century ago and is still used today.

X Rays

X rays were discovered in 1895 by German physicist Wilhelm Conrad Roentgen, the head of the physics department at Würzburg University. Because they were such a mystery to him, Roentgen named them "X rays" when he announced his discovery of their existence. (In mathematics x is used to denote a problem's unknown quantity.) Roentgen's X rays, however, are a form of electromagnetic radiation—of light. They are a form of invisible light with a very short wavelength, shorter than ultraviolet radiation. Because they have much greater energy than visible light or even ultraviolet radiation, X rays can pass through many objects and materials that are opaque to visible light. And it was their penetrating power that made X rays so revolutionary for medical science.

Within days of Roentgen's announcement, doctors began using X rays to look inside the human body. Roentgen himself soon discovered that photographic plates were sensitive to his X rays. That, in turn, meant that it would be possible to take photos of objects that were otherwise hidden from human eyes—for example, the living human skeleton. X rays eventually became the spark for new discoveries and innovations in medicine.

X rays penetrate the body's soft tissues but are absorbed by harder material, such as bone matter. Other dense body tissues will also block or absorb X rays, including cancerous tumors. By exposing a photographic plate sensitive to X rays to an X-ray source, with a part of the body in between the two, doctors can take pictures of the body's internal bones and organs. The photographic negative, called a radiograph, shows bones and dense tissues as light or white regions. The tissues that the X rays passed through easily appear dark. For nearly a hundred years now, doctors have been using these kinds of X-ray images to diagnose diseases, map the location of tumors, detect foreign objects in the body, examine dental cavities, and study damaged or broken bones.

Doctors can also use X rays to study less dense body tissues by first making those tissues opaque to X rays. For example, if a doctor wants to take X rays of a person's gastrointestinal tract, he or she will have the patient first drink a liquid mixture with some material such as barium.

Barium blocks the passage of X rays, so the internal contours of the person's stomach and intestines become visible on a radiograph.

Doctors can also use a process called fluoroscopy to watch certain internal organs in action. The patient stands or lies between an X-ray source and a screen coated with fluorescent material that glows when X rays strike it. A visible image appears when the X rays strike the fluorescent material. An electronic device called an image intensifier brightens the image, which is then displayed on a television monitor.

EEG

While X rays gave rise to the first burst of modern medical imaging technology, another old technique has also been of some use in probing the mysteries of the brain and the mind. A German-American psychiatrist named Hans Berger discovered that he could use small electrical sensors placed on the skull to detect the tiny electrical currents generated by the living brain. In 1929 he put together the first machine capable of doing this and called it an electroencephalograph, or EEG. The word "electroencephalograph" itself is coined from the prefix *electro*, for electricity, and the Greek word *kephalos*, meaning head. Electroencephalography is the amplification, recording, and analysis of these electrical signals. And an electroencephalogram is the tracing or record of this activity as made by the electroencephalograph, or EEG machine.

The neurons in the brain communicate with one another electrochemically; a series of chemical processes sends pulses of electrical potential flowing through neurons. These pulses release neurotransmitter chemicals into the synaptic gap between the axons and dendrites of the neurons. Those chemicals in turn set still more electrical potentials coursing through other neurons—and so on. The result: a continuous set of electrical signals rippling across the surface of the brain as millions of neurons fire, rest, and fire again.

Electrical potential is basically the amount of work it takes to move an electrical charge—an electron—from one point to another. It's measured in the well-known unit of volts. The brain's electrical impulses amount to about 100 microvolts, or .0001 volt. The typical American home has a 120-volt electrical system—more than a million times as much voltage as the brain's electrical impulses.

However, the EEG can detect these minuscule voltage levels. It does so using twenty or so electrodes placed on the head in a set of standardized locations adopted by the International Federation of EEG called the 10/20 system. A cap or harness holds the electrodes in their proper places, and a kind of gluey paste may also be applied to keep them anchored to their particular sites on the skull. The doctor or researcher will carefully measure the location of the electrodes so that subsequent EEGs can be properly compared. Ten pairs of electrodes will then be selected for comparison, their readings sent to the EEG itself.

The EEG actually measures the *difference* between the voltage at these pairs of sites. It can measure the difference in voltage between one pair of electrodes at a time or up to ten pairs at once. Special amplifiers then multiply the voltage differences by up to a million times. The amplified signals then feed into a set of colored pens, which trace them out on a moving strip of paper as a sixteen-channel record of the brain waves. Some EEGs show the signals on an oscilloscope, an instrument that visually displays an electrical wave on a fluorescent screen. Other EEGs store the data in a computer memory for later retrieval and display.

The whole process takes from thirty minutes to an hour. The subject can be asleep; in a relaxed, waking state; or carrying out some kind of restricted activity, such as reading or watching visual stimuli.

The voltage patterns which an EEG detects coming from the brain are called brain waves. Over the years, researchers have been able to identify four main types of brain waves, according to their frequency.

- Beta (β) waves are the highest-frequency brain waves, with frequencies usually between 14 and 30 cycles per second or hertz (abbreviated as Hz, which is the unit of measurement for frequency). They are usually seen in adults and typically are found in the middle and front of the head. They appear related to the brain's sensory and motor-control areas. Beta waves are often seen in people who are sedated with different kinds of tranquilizers.
- Alpha (α) waves, with a frequency of 8–13 hertz, are usually seen in adults who are awake and in a relaxed state. Closing the eyes will enhance the production of alpha waves, while opening the eyes will suppress or desynchronize their patterns. Mental activity or emotional arousal also suppresses alpha waves. On the other hand, bright, flashing lights will often synchronize a person's alpha waves. Their greatest magnitude appears to come from the rear of the

head. Alpha rhythms develop as a person gets older and usually reach maturity when a person is about twelve years old, when they stabilize. They begin declining in frequency and amplitude after age sixty-five.

- Theta (θ) waves are usually seen in children aged two to five. They also replace alpha waves as people become drowsy or enter into light sleep states. Theta waves run from 4 to 7 hertz.
- Delta (δ) waves, from 0.5 to 3 hertz, are the primary brain waves of healthy infants and in the deep sleep of all normal children and adults. When delta waves appear in the EEG records of waking adults, they are almost always associated with some serious medical problems, such as brain tumors.

EEG technology has proved useful in working with people afflicted with epileptic seizures and other kinds of convulsive disorders. These kinds of disorders are caused by abnormal electrical activity in the brain, and an EEG can help map that activity. Also, the advent of today's high-powered desktop computers has made it possible for EEGs to detect *evoked potentials* in brain waves. Evoked potentials are the minuscule voltage changes in the brain's electrical activity that are caused by specific environmental stimuli. When my mother, for example, looks out her bedroom window at the flowers growing in her backyard, her very act of seeing causes a tiny change in voltage in her brain-wave activity. Computerized EEGs can pick out these infinitesimal changes from the welter of background electrical activity in the brain.

However, the EEG has two significant drawbacks for physicians and researchers. First, the bone of the skull happens to effectively block electrical signals; therefore, the EEG, as it is commonly used, cannot produce any kind of detailed map of the brain's electrical activity. A skilled researcher can tell from an EEG tracing that the electrical signal pattern comes from some general part of the brain—the forebrain, for example, or the medulla—but that's about as detailed at it gets. Moreover, an EEG cannot produce "snapshots" of electrical brain activity, images that contain information limited to a few instants of time. Electroencephalograms are essentially "time exposures" and of little help in detailing the moment-to-moment electrical activity in the brain. Only in the last several years have a handful of researchers been able to overcome these serious shortcomings.

CT Scanners

X rays gave doctors an extraordinary new tool for medical diagnosis and treatment. But X-ray technology has its shortcomings. For example, it is very poor at providing images of the body's soft tissues, such as the brain; X rays pass right through these kinds of tissues. Also, X rays can damage the body's tissues by knocking electrons off atoms and giving them an electrical charge—ionizing them. Before this danger was identified, untold thousands of people developed cancer from overexposure to X rays used for medical diagnosis and treating some illnesses. A new form of X-ray process sidesteps those shortcomings and has given physicians a powerful new diagnostic tool. Once called CAT scanning, or computerized axial tomography (the word comes from the Greek root *tomos*, meaning "section" or "slice"), CT (for computerized tomography) scanning combines the old X-ray technology with a new one: computers.

In the early 1970s two researchers more than ten thousand miles apart independently developed the basic principles of the CT scanner. Allan M. Cormack was a physicist in South Africa, and Sir Geoffrey Hounsfield was a British engineer. It was Hounsfield who actually built the first operating model of a CT scanner in 1973. Both Hounsfield and Cormack received the Nobel Prize in 1979 for their work.

X rays produce images of the inside of a human body because, first, they are a very penetrating form of radiation and, second, because some body tissues are more effective at absorbing or blocking X rays than others. With suitable photographic equipment, physicians can create fairly sharp images of the body's internal structure that show bones, organs, and even some rather soft tissue. The CT scanner makes use of this standard X-ray process, but in a rather more sophisticated manner. If one were to pass a series of X-ray beams through a particular part of the body at many different angles, one could make a whole series of radiographs of that particular body section. Each X-ray image would be of that part of the body at a slightly different angle. The problem, of course, is putting all these different images together in a way that makes sense.

Hounsfield and Cormack recognized that the emergence of a new technology would make it possible to combine many two-dimensional X-ray images into a set of three-dimensional "slices" of a human body. And that's what a CT scanner does.

First, the patient lies on a table or gurney that rolls *inside* the CT scanner. The scanner is a tubelike structure that includes a rotating section, or "torus," that looks like a huge doughnut. The doughnut contains the X-ray tube on one side; directly opposite is a set of electronic detectors that "see" the X rays. The moving torus, with its X-ray tube, rotates completely around the patient as he or she lies inside the main body of the scanner. As it does so, a narrow beam of X rays sweeps across the target area of the body. After each short X-ray pulse, the torus moves through another slight angle, and another beam of X rays flashes out.

The detectors on the other side of the rotating torus record the amount of radiation passing through the patient's body. The amount of radiation they detect depends on the density of the bodily tissues that the beam has passed through—each time, with each tiny move of the torus.

The detectors, in turn, send this information to a computer, along with information on the position of the X-ray tube at each particular scan. The computer records, analyzes, and stores the resulting series of X-ray images, each of which has been taken from a different angle. The computer then uses a set of powerful mathematical formulae (in mathematics talk called algorithms) to produce a three-dimensional X-ray image. The resulting picture is like a slice right through the part of the body being examined. Compared to conventional X-ray pictures, the image contains an astonishing amount of detail.

The CT scanner for the first time made it possible to take effective X-ray images of living tissues, such as the human brain, without any discomfort or danger to the patient. The computer-merged combination of individual images provides a much clearer look at the structures within the brain despite the fact that they're made of very soft tissue. Computers can be programmed to highlight areas of an image with different intensity or light levels. Many TV viewers became familiar with the brilliantly colored "false image" pictures of Jupiter and Saturn sent back by the *Voyager 1* and 2 space probes in the 1980s. The computers connected to CT scanners use the same techniques to highlight different structures in the brain. The resulting images are every bit as spectacular as the ones from *Voyager 2*.

They're equally "false," of course. Saturn doesn't really have brilliant blue rings (at least not in visible light), nor is the brain's medulla oblongata really bright yellow in color. However, the ability of computers to manipulate images is what makes CT scanners and the other new medical imaging technologies the effective diagnostic and research tools they are today. Without the computer, none of these imaging machines would exist.

PET SCANS

The success of the CT scanner soon encouraged some researchers to begin looking for other ways to create images of the body's insides in a noninvasive fashion. If computers could be programmed to combine a set of X-ray images into a CT image, certainly they could work similar magic with other techniques. One technique that proved adaptable was tissue autoradiography, which has been used for years to study blood flow and metabolism in animals. In the late 1970s and early 1980s several groups of researchers modified this standard technique into what is today called PET scans.

Tissue autoradiography essentially uses the ability of radioactive materials to "take their own picture." First, a researcher injects an experimental animal with a compound into which has been mixed a radioactive substance called a radioactive isotope, or radioisotope. The radioisotope is chemically identical to normal, nonradioactive substances in the animal's body. So, for example, if the animal's liver uses lots of a particular chemical, the radioisotope version will also accumulate in the same areas of the same organ and in the same concentrations.

When the radioactively labeled compound has had enough time to accumulate in the body part or organ the researcher is studying, the researcher (or, more likely, one of the researcher's assistants) kills the experimental animal and removes the organ in question. The organ is carefully sliced into very thin sections. Then comes the "autoradiography" part. The researcher lays the individual slices on a piece of film that is sensitive to radioactivity. This is usually some form of X-ray film. The researcher's X-ray film records the distribution of the radioactively labeled compound in each tissue slice. The result? A set of images of how the radioisotope is distributed in the sample and thus some information about the organ's functions.

By using different kinds of radioactive compounds, researchers can uncover different types of information about the organ or tissue they are studying. This is because the body uses different compounds for different uses. Glucose, for example, is particularly useful in studying the brain's metabolism because this form of sugar is the primary source of food for neurons.

Researchers who had been using tissue autoradiography were quite taken by the CT-scanner breakthrough. They realized that it might be possible to reconstruct the distribution of a radioisotope in a particular part of the body the same way the CT scanner reconstructs an organ's anatomy using X-ray images. The key would be to measure the radioactive emissions coming from the body tissue or section in question.

One problem researchers faced was finding a way to actually create maps of organs and other tissues using radioactivity. They solved the problem by identifying a group of radioactive isotopes that emit positrons. These are subatomic particles that are identical to electrons, except that they have a positive charge rather than a negative one. They are, in fact, a form of antimatter.

When a positron encounters a "normal" electron, the two annihilate each other. And because electrons are a part of every normal atom of matter, this happens almost immediately after the radioisotope releases a positron. When an electron and positron annihilate each other, they release two gamma rays at a specific energy level. The two gamma rays almost always head off in nearly opposite directions. This, in turn, means that a set of detectors placed around the positron-emitting object can easily "backtrack" the gamma rays to their point of origin, which means that one can map the location of the radioisotope in a sample. To medical researchers, this means they can "see" which areas of the body are using particular positron-emitting versions of otherwise normal elements or chemicals. They can also map the amount of a compound used by measuring how much gamma-ray energy is emitted. Researchers can even track the movements of positron-emitting compounds as they move into and through different regions of the body. It is the positron-emitting nature of these radioactive compounds that gives PET its name.

Another problem faced by researchers was that radioisotopes are radioactive. Some radioactivity is practically harmless. Alpha particles are nothing more than the nuclei of helium atoms and can't even pass through a sheet of paper. Beta radiation is really a stream of electrons and is also easily blocked. However, X rays and gamma rays are more powerful forms of electromagnetic radiation, and it can take a considerable amount of shielding to stop their penetration. Gamma rays can knock electrons from their positions around atoms, ionizing the atoms and giving them an electrical charge. Strong enough gamma radiation can even break apart the nuclei of atoms, turning them into radioactive elements that themselves may emit gamma rays as they decay.

The solution was to use positron-emitting radioisotopes with very short half-lives. The radioisotopes most commonly used today in PET scans include carbon 11, nitrogen 13, oxygen 15, and fluorine 18. These isotopes have half-lives measured in minutes rather than days or years or centuries. A typically sized sample used for a PET scan study will have decayed completely into nonradioactivity in less than an hour. And because they are chemically identical to their nonradioactive siblings, researchers can use them to label natural compounds and drugs without changing any chemical or biological properties. This is what makes it possible to use the methods, knowledge, and interpretation of more traditional tissue autoradiography to be applied to humans in PET scanning.

Fluorine 18 is particularly useful for some kinds of PET-scan experiments. It has a half-life of only 110 minutes, so it poses no radiation hazard to the patient. More to the point, fluorine 18 can take the place of oxygen atoms in molecules of glucose, one of the brain's main sources of energy. PET scans can then pinpoint which parts of the brain are working the hardest during certain functions—such as thinking a thought, silently reading a word, or experiencing an emotion—by "seeing" the areas of the brain that are using a lot of glucose.

Another useful isotope for PET is oxygen 15. This radioactive isotope of oxygen has a half-life of only two minutes, and an entire sample of oxygen 15 will have decayed into a nonradioactive isotope in about ten minutes. Researchers can substitute oxygen 15 for nonradioactive versions of oxygen in molecules of water—good old H_2O. They can then inject the labeled water into a person's vein. In about one minute the radioactive water will be carried into the brain by the bloodstream. Researchers can then use PET scans to track blood flow in the brain, which gives them another way of measuring which areas of the brain are more active than others.

MRI

In 1973, the same year that Geoffrey Hounsfield was building the first CT scanner, physicians in Great Britain began using another mechanical offspring of physics and computer science for medical diagnosis. Nuclear magnetic resonance (NMR) had long been used by physicists to study tiny samples of various compounds. Medical researchers found a way to transmogrify this obscure and abstruse physics technique into a powerful new tool for imaging the insides of the human body, including the human brain. In the process, they also carried out a bit of public-relations magic.

A still-popular conception of atoms pictures them as tiny solar systems. Just as the sun is at the center of our solar system and the planets revolve around it, the nucleus lies at the center of an atom, and the electrons orbit around it. This description is not really correct. Atoms are actually so strange that it's hard to talk about what is "real" when one is talking about them. But the analogy can actually be pushed a little further.

Many of the planets in the solar system (including Earth) and the sun itself have magnetic fields, with clearly defined north and south magnetic poles. The nuclei of atoms also have their own tiny magnetic fields. What's more, with the right equipment one can get the nuclei of many atoms to line up magnetically and even resonate or vibrate together. Ergo, "nuclear magnetic resonance."

Medical researchers realized that they could use this characteristic of atomic nuclei to create images of various organs, including the brain. They also eventually stumbled upon the fact that, these days, the word "nuclear" carries a lot of negative connotations. NMR has nothing to do with radioactivity, but that word "nuclear" was disturbing and even intimidating for many people. So the name was changed to protect the innocent. NMR imaging eventually became *magnetic resonance imaging*, or MRI.

An MRI scanner is an incredibly clever piece of machinery that uses magnets and radio waves to turn the atoms inside a person's body into tiny radio transmitters. The patient lies on a gurney that slides him or her into the tubelike scanner. MRI scanners, PET scanners, and CT scanners all look very much alike. However, the MRI scanner does not use X rays. Instead, the patient is surrounded by curved panels containing coils that produce radio signals. Surrounding the coils are a series of ring-shaped electromagnets cooled to nearly absolute zero by liquid helium. The electromagnets produce a magnetic field that's thirty thousand times stronger than Earth's magnetic field. Needless to say, patients with metal plates in their heads are not candidates for MRI scans. The MRI's incredibly powerful magnetic field would rip the metal plate right out of the person's skull.

The atomic nuclei inside the atoms that make up a person's body tissues are like tiny magnets with north and south poles. Ordinarily, they randomly point in a myriad different directions. The nuclei are also spinning* around an axis, which, like Earth's, is not necessarily the same as their magnetic axis. When the electromagnets are turned on, the immensely powerful magnetic field acts to align the magnetic axes of all the nuclei so that their north and south magnetic poles are pointing in the same direction. They continue to spin in various directions, however. The magnetic field also causes the nuclei to vibrate at a specific frequency. Now the atomic nuclei are acting like tiny radios, sending and receiving radio signals.

Next, the MRI scanner sends out its own powerful pulse of radio waves from its radio coils. The pulse is aimed at the particular part of the body to be imaged—such as the brain. The radio pulse knocks the magnetic axes of the nuclei out of alignment so that they are no longer lined up with the MRI's own electromagnetic field. At the same time, the radio pulse forces the *spin axes* of the atomic nuclei to all line up together and *spin* coherently.

When the radio pulse stops after a few instants, the magnetic poles of the nuclei snap back into alignment with the MRI's powerful magnetic field. As they do so, they all send out their own faint burst of radio signals.

The MRI scanner's detectors receive those radio signals, amplify them, digitize them, and send them on to the scanner's computer. As the radio signals pass through intervening tissue and bone, their strength and duration change. The computer uses a sophisticated program that takes this information and turns it into an image of the body part being scanned.

CT scanning is particularly good at imaging soft tissue like the brain and its internal structures. This makes it useful in detecting the areas of the brain affected by injuries, tumors, hemorrhages, and strokes. MRI scans are very helpful in imaging areas in the head where hard and soft tissue meet, in looking at the spinal cord, and in imaging areas of the brain affected by strokes that CT scans may not see as clearly. MRI also does a better job than CT of creating high-resolution images of the brain's gray and white matter. This makes it particularly useful in imaging some disorders that affect nerve fibers, such as multiple sclerosis.

---

*Sort of; kind of. Atomic "spin" is another one of those difficult-to-explain physics things.

Unlike the X rays used in CT scans and the gamma rays detected in PET scans, magnetic fields and radio waves are perfectly harmless. It is the nuclei of the atoms in the body themselves that produce the signals that the MRI scanner detects and turns into images.

There can be some discomfort associated with getting an MRI scan. The operation of the electromagnets and the radio coils is very noisy, so the patient must have a good set of earplugs. It is also often necessary for the person being scanned to lie perfectly still, especially if the image being made is of an organ like the brain. So the patient may get a mild sedative. Finally, like PET and CT scanners, the working cavity of many MRI scanners is very narrow and confining and can be quite uncomfortable for people who are claustrophobic. However, the actual scan itself is not uncomfortable at all. In fact, the person being scanned doesn't feel a thing.

DURING THE EARLY DAYS of photography in the nineteenth century, people had to stand perfectly still for many minutes while the camera lens remained open. Photographic plates were not very sensitive to light and needed long exposure times to produce a passable image. In somewhat similar fashion, CT scans generally require long "exposure times" to create an image. Their temporal resolutions are measured in multiples of minutes.

PET scans are like the generation of cameras created by such pioneers as George Eastman. Those cameras used photographic film that was much more sensitive to light. The camera shutter needed to be open for only a second or less to get a good picture. For the first time, the man and woman on the street could take pictures good enough to keep and share with others. "Snapshots" came into existence, and Eastman (of Kodak fame) started a new industry. In somewhat the same way, the first generation of PET scans had temporal resolutions measured in minutes. Today's generation of PET scanners can take computer-massaged snapshots with time frames measured in seconds.

Then there are MRI scans. Today's still cameras take pictures with exposure times measured in hundredths of a second. Movie cameras take dozens of frames per second, and when run through a projector, they create the illusion of seamless movement. The early generations of MRI scanners had temporal resolutions measured in seconds. Now a new form of the technology, called functional MRI, or fMRI, can take millisecond snapshots of processes going on in the living human brain.

By taking a series of these fMRI images, researchers can now create computer-generated "movies" of the brain in action—thinking, reading, seeing, speaking, dreaming. For example, a researcher using fMRI can follow the process by which different parts of the brain work together as a person sees a word and silently speaks it. And the researcher can do this while the subject is actually carrying out the task at hand.

THESE REMARKABLE new imaging machines, along with some others we will soon encounter, are opening vistas of knowledge to brain researchers. They are giving us new insights into how the brain grows from infancy to adulthood; how it governs our body's movements and senses; how it learns and remembers; how and where it generates emotions; how it makes, stores, and uses the method of communication called language; how it sometimes breaks down or falls apart; and even how it creates that mysterious reality we call "mind."

PART II

MAPPING THE BRAIN

What seas what shores what gray rocks and what islands
What water lapping the bow
And scent of pine and the woodthrush singing through the fog
What images return
O my daughter.
—T.S. Eliot, "Marina"

CHAPTER 4

THE GROWING BRAIN

My MOTHER has been playing the piano for as long as I can remember. When my family still consisted of only me and my parents, they bought their first home, one of the first tract houses in Camarillo, California. Not long after that, they purchased a piano, and she began playing again. "I must have been about fifteen years old when I first learned to play," she recalls today. "We had been in New York City for about three years then, after leaving Hungary."

She pauses a moment, going back in memory. "It was a long time ago, and it's a little hazy, but I recall that we had an upright piano in our apartment in the Bronx. My dad would drive my sister and me to our music lessons. It was a woman who taught us"—She corrects herself. "No. I remember now. It was some kind of music school, a little school, just a few kids; that's where your Aunt Edie and I had our lessons. We only took them for about a year. That's all the training I ever had." She laughs.

Ten years later, after leaving the Bronx and that piano behind and taking a cross-country trip from New York City to Los Angeles in the middle of World War II; after three years at UCLA and a romance with a young sailor back from the Pacific that turned into a marriage; after her first child and her first home, my mother started playing the piano again. She was a little rusty at first, but soon it all came back to her. For the next thirty years, as long as there were still children in the family home in Ventura, California, my mother would periodically sit down at the upright piano in the dining room, take out some sheet music, sight-read, and play.

Bob Dylan once wrote that "those not busy being born are busy dying." The truth is, the body does both. Our bodies are constantly busy dying and being born. Nearly every cell dies off, only to be replaced by new ones. The one dramatic exception to this rule is the nervous system, particularly the brain. By the time we are four or five years old, our brains have finished creating neurons. The 100 billion or so we have at that point are all that we'll ever have.

My mother was older than most children are when they begin playing a musical instrument like the piano. Even at fifteen, however, her brain was capable of learning something new and retaining that knowledge. It had probably been years since a single new neuron had been born in her brain. But the ones she had then—and still has—created the new pathways necessary for mastering the new task.

The brain is an amazing organ, especially when it is trained early. Brain researchers have long accepted the fact that the brain of a newborn baby grows fast and furiously. It was also "common knowledge" in the neurosciences that much of the brain's neuronal circuitry was hardwired, set in place at a fairly early age. Only in the last couple of decades have researchers begun to learn just how sophisticated the growth and maturation of the infant brain really is. And it is only in the last few years that old assumptions about the hardwired brain have been overturned.

FROM CONCEPTION TO BIRTH

Twenty-five years ago, brain scientists already had some ideas about how the brain forms during embryonic and fetal development. That knowledge, though, was woefully small. In the last several years researchers have learned about a whole array of molecules that act as cues, or triggers, for the brain's development and growth. The entire sequence of fetal development, from fertilized egg to birth, is controlled and timed by the release of these specific proteins and other chemical compounds. These chemical gurus of fetal development are in turn controlled, turned on and off, by various genes in the human genetic code. Researchers are only now beginning to uncover the first tiny hints of where those genes are and what they do. Still unanswered are the questions of how and why these developmental genes can turn on only when needed and turn off—forever—when finished.

The first glimmerings of the brain and nervous system begin to appear just two weeks after conception. The cells that make up the new human embryo start to separate into different structures. One is a layer of cells called the ectoderm. Some of the cells in the ectoderm soon begin to form a flat sheet called the neural plate, from which the brain and nervous system will develop. From the neural plate grow the cells that will become the brain, and nervous system. A protein called nerve growth factor (NGF), along with instructions from regulatory genes and chemical signals from nearby cells, cause some of them to begin developing into glial cells, the "scaffolding" for the brain's neurons.

In fact, the embryo begins to develop from the inside out. The central nervous system begins to develop first, and the rest of the body forms around this neural core. The neural plate curls into a cylinder called the neural tube. The neural tube will develop into the brain, spinal cord, and entire nervous system.

Neurons begin developing at an accelerated rate. The nascent brain now generates some 250,000 neurons *per minute*, continuously, for the next nine months. Hundreds of billions of neurons are created, and a good 50 percent of them are killed off. Various hormones and other chemicals pare away unneeded neurons, just as a whittler with a switchblade carves wood shavings from a stick. What is left is the finished scaffolding of the newborn baby's brain. At this point the embryo is still so small that the human eye can barely see it. Yet it already contains within itself the instructions to create eyes and the brain that will use them to see the outer world.

By the time the embryo is twenty-five days old, the neural tube has started to bend into a curve. The scaffolding cells (the glia) begin spreading out like the spokes of a wheel. The new neurons then develop, migrating outward along the glia like pioneers following wagon-wheel tracks into new territory. Some chemicals attract the neurons along the appropriate pathways. Others act like little chemical magnets, pushing the neurons forward.

Once the neurons at the front end of the still-developing neural tube have found their rightful place in the world, their job is only half-done. Now they begin producing dendrites and axons. Dendrites are the short treelike extensions from the neuron's body. They are somewhat like the antennae that receive electrochemical signals from other neurons. Axons are the single, long fibers that extend from each neuron and act as the "broadcast towers" that send signals to other nerve cells. The synapses are the tiny gaps where data transmission takes place between axons and dendrites. Once again, the developing brain uses special chemical molecules to guide the dendrites and axons to their correct locations. Some molecules act like signposts or traffic cops, staying in one location and directing the traffic. Other molecules travel up and down the neural roadways like trail guides, finding the growing axons and bringing them along the correct path. Still other chemicals are stop signs or directional signals, telling the axons and dendrites to halt or move in another direction.

Less than three weeks have passed since conception, but already the basic architecture of the brain is being laid down in lines of living flesh. At thirty-five days after conception, the embryo is both the shape and size of this capital C. The neural tube starts to develop three distinct swellings at the top of the C. These minuscule bulges will begin to develop into the three main parts of the brain: the forebrain, midbrain, and hindbrain. The rest of the C will become the spinal cord.

By the time another two weeks have passed, the foremost swelling in the neural tube begins to dominate the structure. The emerging shape of the brain and spinal cord, and to a lesser degree the beginnings of the peripheral nervous system, can now be seen. The protoforebrain will soon begin to develop into the two distinct cerebral hemispheres of the brain.

The axons of some neurons in the developing brain may reach their destinations by aiming not at the final target but at intermediate ones. When NASA scientists launched the Voyager 2 spacecraft in 1976, they did not aim it directly at the planet Neptune, its final destination. Instead, Voyager first traveled to Jupiter, where it used that planet's gravitational force to slingshot it to Saturn. From Saturn the space probe traveled to Uranus, and then finally to Neptune. In somewhat analogous fashion, axons in the developing fetal brain may make several stops along the way to their final destination.

Carla J. Shatz, a neurobiologist at Stanford University, has uncovered a striking example of this process. Shatz studies the development of the neurons that carry signals from the eyes to the visual cortex at the back of the brain. The visual cortex is the area of the brain that processes information coming from the eyes. These fibers must first make connections in a part of the brain called the visual thalamus. Then axons from the visual thalamus must reach out to connect with a part of the visual cortex that brain researchers call layer four. During fetal development, these axons arrive at their destination before visual-layer four has itself come into existence. It's a bit like an arrow reaching the space where the bull's-eye will be before anyone has even set up the target.

Shatz and her colleagues have found that certain short-lived cells act as "intermediate targets" during fetal development. Neurobiologists had long known of the existence of these cells (called subplate neurons) but had always assumed they had no particular function. Shatz and her associates showed otherwise. In a series of experiments, they removed these cells from the brains of cat fetuses early in the fetal-development process. They found that the axons from the visual thalamus would wander about in the region below the visual cortex, never connecting to the cortex itself. When she removed these intermediate target neurons later in the cats' fetal development, the cats' visual cortexes did not develop properly. They didn't possess the structures needed to tell the difference between visual stimuli from the left and right eyes. Shatz has been quoted as saying that in the former experiment "the axons can't find the right city. If we get rid of them later, the axons don't find the right address."

AT AROUND FOUR to four and a half months into pregnancy, the fetus has finished its primary brain-building tasks. The axons have all pretty much reached their main locations. Like a house whose wooden frame is now finished, the brain of the embryo has its main structures in place. The first phase of the brain's development is over. The second is about to begin.

Imagine that you are building a telephone system from scratch. First, you must string the main telephone cables that connect major locations, like cities and towns. Once that's done, you must connect each of the people in each of the cities to one another. Even then, your job is not completed. Now you must make sure that the telephone lines do in fact go to the right locations and that you've got all the phone numbers correctly assigned. This is the task that the neurons in the brain of the fetus now begin to perform. The way they do it is both simple and startling.

They begin firing. Spontaneously. The neurons are in a sense trying to make sure that they really are connected to the right location, that they're reaching the right party at the other end of the line. It's as if you started autodialing each number in your new phone book until someone responded. If someone answers, and it's the right person, you can confirm that the connection is a good one. If the wrong person answers, you may either have to change the phone number or perhaps even take out the entire phone line. (No, this isn't what real phone companies do. This is an analogy, and by now it's being stretched pretty thin.) In the same way, the neuronal pathways that are good, correct, proper, useful, get reinforced. The ones that aren't, don't. They eventually disappear as the neurons involved weaken and die.

At first, this process goes on without any external stimuli. For example, the neurons that make up the visual-perception system in the brain begin testing themselves before the fetal eyes have even developed the cells needed for vision. As pregnancy progresses through the second and into the third trimester, the fetus's sensory organs begin to mature enough to detect outside stimuli even from within the womb. The fetus starts to respond to detectable light levels and to sound. Yes, it really can hear Pachelbel's "Canon" when Mom holds the tape player next to her belly. The brain also starts sending commands through the developing motor nerves to the fetal legs and hands. The fetus begins to move in response, testing its muscles and strengthening the neural circuits.

By the time the infant is born, nine months after conception, its brain has been thoroughly tested and prepped for life outside the womb. All the essential circuits have been laid down, and the brain is still growing neurons at an astonishing rate. It will continue to do so for a few more years. But by now it's not the number of neurons that count.

It's the number of connections.

THE MALLEABLE BRAIN

When cognitive scientists talk about the developing brains of newborns and infants, they frequently use the words "malleable" or "neuroplasticity." They are good descriptions of the growing human brain. While we are young, our brains are like lumps of clay in the hands of a master sculptor or a fresh canvas waiting for the painter's brush strokes. The sculptor molds the clay into the shape she wants. But if she changes her mind or has a new flash of inspiration, she can push and pull the clay into a slightly different shape or create a whole new object.

Similarly, a painter can create a landscape that looks just so and then, a few hours or days later, change that mountain from snowy to tree-covered or add a lake in the foreground. He can even paint a whole new scene over the old one—assuming he is creating an oil or acrylic painting and not a watercolor. Many of the paintings by the great Renaissance masters actually have other, older images hidden beneath the visible one.

In somewhat the same way, the brain of a newborn baby is a rough-ly shaped lump of clay waiting to be perfected or a sketched-out paint-ing waiting to be filled in and finished. The infant brain isn't a blank canvas; the analogy doesn't stretch that far. Each of us is born with a brain that already has a remarkably complex structure and regions that are already functioning. But as soon as we've been jerked into the cold, bright reality of the delivery room, we begin experiencing and process-ing a flood of new information. Since the early and mid-1980s, researchers using the new imaging technologies have begun learning just how furiously the brain works to process all the new information and how that work changes the very structure of the brain itself.

Positron-emission tomography (PET) has given researchers a dra-matic new look at the changes in organization that the human brain goes through between birth and adulthood. PET scans can track the pattern of glucose use in the brain. As mentioned earlier, glucose is a form of sugar that constitutes the brain's main sources of energy. It is the arche-typal "brain food." By substituting radioactive isotopes of oxygen or car-bon for nonradioactive atoms in glucose, researchers can use PET to track where and how the brain uses this energy source as it works. As the structure of the brain changes during its early growth and matura-tion, these patterns of glucose metabolism also change.

While not particularly startling or amazing—this is not fodder for the weekly tabloids—the results of these kinds of studies do shed new light on how the brain grows itself into adulthood. The data on patterns of glucose use by the brain clearly show a relationship between a meta-bolic increase within certain brain structures and the simultaneous emergence of certain behaviors and brain functions.

One of the first researchers to use PET scans to track the way the brain grows from infancy through childhood was Dr. Harold Chugani. Director of the PET Center at the Children's Hospital of Michigan, Chugani was working at the University of California at Los Angeles in the 1980s as PET began being used extensively in brain research. Chugani studied people afflicted with intractable epilepsy. The standard drugs used to control their seizures had not worked. The only recourse these patients had was surgery to remove the portion of the brain that was triggering the seizures. Chugani was using PET scans to try and pin-point the offending brain-seizure sites.

At the same time, he was able to note which areas of the brain were most active by their levels of glucose metabolism. As Chugani examined the glucose use of people ranging from infants to adults, he began to see the developmental timetable for various regions of the brain.

For example, in infants younger than five weeks old, glucose use is highest in the areas of the brain that control the body's basic processes. One such area is the sensorimotor cortex, a strip of brain tissue that runs from left to right across the top of the brain. Another is the brain stem, located at the base of the brain, where the spinal cord begins. At the same time, a newborn baby's cerebral cortex has relatively low levels of glucose use. A newborn baby cannot talk, read, carry out complex mental computations, or spin elaborate fantasies about alien life on other planets. These are all "higher order" mental functions that involve the brain's cerebral cortex. In fact, a newborn cannot even control its bowel movements. But an infant *can* grab a pipe or stick and hold on for dear life. This grasping reflex—a handy survival trick under some circumstances—is one of several such reflexes controlled by the brain stem. Brain function in newborns is mostly limited to these so-called primary sensory and motor areas. This pattern of infant behavior is reflected in the colorful PET images of their brains.

By the time an infant is about three months old, though, glucose use is beginning to take place throughout much of the cerebral cortex. Areas deep in the brain that are essential for coordinated movement (like walking) begin to show high levels of glucose use. The sensorimotor cortex uses more and more sugar fuel as it becomes more and more active. At the same time, the seemingly random leg and arm movements are being replaced by more coordinated motions. The infant starts reaching for objects—Mother's earrings, Dad's finger, Grandma Toni's hair. Meanwhile, the area at the front of the brain—the frontal cortex—and other regions usually involved in creating abstract concepts remain less metabolically active than the rest of the brain.

By the time the infant is eight to nine months old, and sometimes even earlier, some cognitive development has begun. Most infants are babbling, a clear precursor to their first words and phrases. They already are beginning to connect abstract concepts like "Mommy" and "cat" with specific persons and animals. Sure enough, PET images now begin to reveal increased use of glucose—and thus higher metabolism or working levels—in the areas of the brain intimately involved in thought, speech, and concepts. These include the frontal cortex and other brain areas known as the association cortexes. In these images,

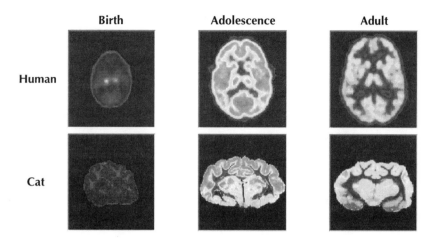

FIG. 4.1.   These PET images show the remarkable similarities in brain glucose metabolism between humans and cats at the same developmental stages in their lives.

then, we begin to actually "see" the emergence of conscious thought and self-awareness.

By the time the young child is a year old, images of the brain made with PET scanners begin to resemble those of normal older children and adults. The most active regions in these images are those involved in visual perception, emotions, and higher cognitive functions, such as thinking and language. At age four, a child's brain is more than twice as active metabolically as that of an adult, consuming glucose at an astonishing rate. This metabolic brainstorm continues until the child is around ten years old and then begins to slow down. The brain's use of glucose plateaus at adult levels around age sixteen.

Another way of learning more about how the human brain grows and develops is to compare PET maps of the human brain with those of an animal, such as a cat (Fig. 4.1). Researchers who have carried out PET scans of the brains of young and mature house cats have found significant parallels between glucose metabolic rates in the cats' brains and the development of standard catlike behavior patterns. This is just what researchers studying human infants have found as well. So it is now possible to determine when a particular region or system in the young brain approaches maturity by detecting when its rate of glucose use begins to drop from earlier high levels.

5 days   **6 years**   **Adult**

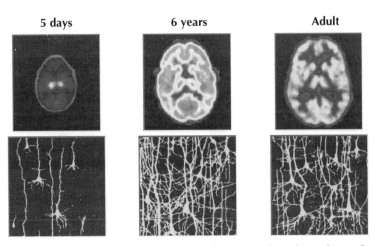

FIG. 4.2.   This set of images reveals the "why" as well as the "what" of active glucose use in the growing human brain. The PET scans at the top show the highest levels of brain activity in humans five days old, six years old, and in adulthood. The images depict the density of the connections among neurons in the brain. In newborns a typical brain region will have relatively few neuron interconnections. But by the time the child is six years old, the brain has developed a massive network of synaptic connections among its neurons. In adults, those neural networks have already been "pruned down" somewhat, since neuron connections that are rarely used get discarded.

The "why" of these remarkable images of elevated brain activity at different ages is directly related to the patterns of growth of the brain's structures and complexity. Figure 4.2 compares PET scans showing the relative glucose metabolic rate at three different ages. The drawings beneath the PET scans show the relative complexity of brain structure at each age. Anatomic studies reveal that the increases in glucose usage by different structures or regions during brain development happen at the same time that the brain's neurons develop more and more connections with one another. At the same time, the density of capillaries—the tiny blood vessels that carry blood to every cell in the body—also increases in the human frontal cortex.

As Harold Chugani and other researchers have found, the growing brain must maintain the many trillions of synaptic connections among neurons. We are all born with pretty much the same number of neurons in our brains that we will have for most of our lives. Children do not grow more brain cells after about age four, nor do they lose them. (At least not in childhood. Brain cells do start dying off as we reach old age, even in people without any brain diseases.)

What does change are *the number of connections* among the brain neurons. It's the connections that count. In fact, researchers now know that the brains of normal growing children have at least twice as many synapses as those of adults. Very early in our lives, our brains grow far more synaptic connections than they really need. Each connection between and among neurons, each synaptic pathway, represents a possible road that an electrochemical impulse may travel. The pathways that get repeatedly used get selectively strengthened. Those that do not get used, or used only rarely, will eventually be physically eliminated and disappear from the brain for good.

Some brain pathways are indeed "hardwired" in at birth. Billions of years of evolution have created a set of instructions in the human genetic code that provide for a whole set of predetermined pathways for the brain. All of the basic body functions, for example, are hardwired into the brain. We don't have to practice breathing, sleeping, hearing, seeing, or smelling. We do not have to learn how to suck (the sucking reflex for breast-feeding) or how to grasp our tiny fists together (that grasping reflex so helpful to primates that once lived in forests). Nor do we have to learn how to make the noises—crying, whining, gurgling, snorting, clicking— that will within months metaphorphosize into spoken language.

Once an infant's brain has matured enough to start controlling facial muscles, he or she will begin to smile. Smiling, though, is not learned. It is a facial behavior that is hardwired into the brain. It appears at the same time in all humans, no matter what their racial background or geographic location.

THE ACTUAL TIMETABLE for the development of different brain regions also seems to be genetically predetermined. What is not hardwired into the brain is how intensively each region or structure will develop. It is at this point that "nurture" begins to guide the development of "nature." Michael Phelps of UCLA, one of the developers of the PET scan, has said: "The thing that determines which connections are saved is education in the broadest sense. . . . If we teach our children early enough, it will affect the 'wiring' of their brains."

One way of looking at the role of education or external environmental stimulation for the growing brain is to look at the other side of the coin. What happens when an infant brain is *deprived* of stimuli?

Once again, the common house cat has provided us with a powerful and disturbing answer. In the 1950s neurobiologists David Hubel of Harvard University and Torsten Wiesel of Rockefeller University carried out some pioneering studies of vision and the brain's visual cortex. They used cats in those studies and later won the Nobel Prize for their work.

In one set of experiments Hubel and Wiesel covered the eyes of cats during certain periods of their infancy. Once they removed the blindfolds, they discovered that the cats still could not see. Their eyes were fine, but the neurons that created the connections between their eyes and their visual cortex were impaired. Because those particular pathways had not been used at a critical time during their brain's development, they did not mature. The cats were permanently blind.

Another more tragic negative example can be found in the stories and studies of so-called wolf children. The medical literature contains several documented cases of children who were somehow abandoned early in life and were raised in the wild by animals such as wolves. Rudyard Kipling's famous story of Mowgli was based on anecdotal tales of such children. In every documented case of such a child, two important facts stand out. None of the children possess language skills when they are discovered and brought back to human civilization. Moreover, none of them are ever able to gain such skills. Like the kittens permanently deprived of sight, human wolf children are permanently deprived of language.

And for the same reason. As we will learn in more detail later on, language is a brain-based skill that every normal child begins developing shortly after birth. The essential skills for both spoken and signed languages are in place by the time an infant is eighteen to thirty months old. If a child has not been exposed to language and begun practicing those skills by the time he or she is three to four years hold, the child will *never* possess normal language. Language skills reside in the brain and in the neuronal connections within the brain. Those connections are most easily laid down early in life, when the brain is still highly malleable. The older we get, the harder it is for us to learn a second language—and a first language, too, for that matter.

On the more positive side, our own experience provides evidence for the importance of environmental enrichment to the growing brain. For example, infants or young children who do learn a second or third language will speak like natives. They will *think* in the language without having to do translations in their heads. Again, the reason is that the neural pathways that encode the language are created and strengthened during a time when the brain is still very malleable.

In a typical computer, the microcircuits and wiring have been built in advance. There they are, literally hardwired, and they don't change. The programs run on our computers, however, can and do change. Windows 3.0, Windows 3.1, Windows 95—each is a new and different version of an earlier program. Someone—usually a lot of someones—have rewritten the code for the program. The software developers have added new features, improved other features, fixed bugs, and probably added a few undocumented tricks. In many cases the programmers even hide their names somewhere in the program. Think of the hardwired circuitry of the "box" as the basic structural shell of a house. The computer programs are the carpeting, furniture, appliances, paint, and wallpaper.

The human brain also has a basic architectural structure. That structure starts being fashioned during the first weeks of an embryo's life. It is essentially finished by the time a child is four or five years old. But there remains much that can be done even after that point.

BRAIN PLASTICITY AND EDUCATION

Our increasing knowledge of the growing brain and its remarkable malleability has some practical implications for how we teach our children. Repeated stimulation strengthens existing synaptic connections among brain cells and activates the creation of new connections. Chugani has therefore suggested that "it's better to expose a kid to a lot of things over a period of years rather than trying to cover subjects one at a time in brief, intensive workshops."

In fact, it appears that much current instruction in today's schools is based on a premise with no foundation. Most educational theorists have assumed that children need to get some kind of immediate feedback or reward for getting the "right answer." Instruction in everything from arithmetic to world history is broken down into bite-sized pieces, with answers available at every little step of the way. In the real world, however, the brain is much more complicated and sophisticated than educators have assumed. As we'll see later in more detail, the brain does a lot more than just learn by drill and practice. It has many small modules or neural networks that are constantly operating in parallel. It would make a lot more sense—brain sense, anyway—to present children with plenty of problems that don't have any immediate, simple solutions. Then, as the children work over longer periods of time at trying to solve the problems and find some answers, they strengthen their brain's existing neural connections and also growing new ones. The result will be knowledge that the children will retain for a much longer time than they would if they'd simply memorized the "right" answer.

At the same time, it is important not to push children too hard. We have all heard of the well-meaning but overcompetitive parents who try to get little Nancy to start learning calculus at age six or who send little Billy to violin camp at age three. That kind of excessive educational pushing can cause levels of anxiety in the child leading to the release of stress hormones. And those kinds of body chemicals can actually destroy neurons.

THE GREAT WINDOW of learning opportunity for the human brain clearly appears during the childhood years, especially up to about age ten. But that doesn't mean that we—or our brains—are over the hill after that point. My mother, remember, first learned how to play the piano when she was fifteen and took lessons for only a year. She can still sight-read music today, nearly sixty years later. In fact, it doesn't matter how old our brains are—fifteen, twenty-five, or fifty years old, or more. As long as we stay healthy and active, the brain will retain some of its plasticity, growing more dendrites and axons and forging new connections among them.

CHAPTER 5

WALKING THE WALK

MY BROTHER TIM is about a year old and just starting to walk. He takes a few steps in the living room of our new home near Ventura—and falls. He laughs; he cries. He tries again. "Come here! Over here," my father urges him, smiling encouragingly. Tim tries again. One, two, three, steps. He falls. Then again, a few awkward steps, and he makes it to my dad's outstretched arms. We all cheer.

My mother turns to me and says, "You know, you didn't start walking until you were nearly two years old." I am surprised and embarrassed. Good grief, I was so *slow*. "In fact," she continues, "you hardly even crawled. You would scoot your way around on the floor on your rear end, pushing yourself along." My dad laughs good-naturedly and obviously agrees.

"But when you did start walking," my mother concludes, "you *did* it. Just like that."

Well, maybe I was slow getting started, but by God I at least skipped the preliminaries. Sort of.

Today a researcher with an MRI (magnetic resonance imaging) scanner could tell my mother precisely what parts of my two-year-old brain would have been actively working when I was moving my leg or my foot or when I flexed the fingers of my left hand as I reached to grasp a spoon at breakfast. Even back in 1950, when I first started walking, brain researchers had a pretty good idea which brain areas controlled which parts of the body. But now the new imaging technologies are casting new light on the brain's motor-control functions. With a clarity never before achieved, we can now observe what our brain is doing when we play a guitar, catch a fly ball, or react to a red light as we're driving down a city street.

One of the people who is making great strides in this area is a researcher in San Francisco who has given new life to an old imaging technology, the electroencephalogram (EEG).

THE SOUPED-UP EEG

Alan Gevins is director of the EEG Systems Laboratory in San Francisco. His office and lab facilities are in a beautiful new building that borders the Embarcadero Plaza. A double-decker freeway that was smashed by the 1989 Loma Prieta earthquake has been torn down and bulldozed away, revealing a gorgeous view of San Francisco Bay. On the autumn day I visited with Gevins, skateboarders were zipping through the plaza, and crowds of people during the lunch hour browsed and shopped at an outdoor crafts fair.

Up in the conference room in the EEG Systems office, Gevins leaned forward at the table and talked about his journey into EEG technology, old and new, and his fascination with the brain.

Gevins's interest in the brain was sparked when he was eighteen and a student at MIT. While he was there, he did a thesis on the effects of electromagnetic fields in the brain.

"I have had really great teachers," he said. "I was really lucky. I studied with Marvin Minsky in artificial intelligence and with Jerry Letvin, the guy who discovered feature detectors in the brain before Hubel and Wiesel. And with Meld and Hein, the guys who had the glasses where people saw upside down, and the kittens, who both saw the same things—one was passive; one was active. So I got to carry on the tradition of neurocybernetics to the next generation. I chose to study brain waves, EEGs, because they are the most direct signal of the actual real-time functioning of the brain."

When Gevins turned twenty-six, he came to the Langley Porter Neuropsychiatric Institute, located at the University of California Medical School in San Francisco. Two years later, in 1974, he became the lab's director—the second director in the lab's history. His experiences over the next several years were not exactly sweetness and light.

"I'd get a dollar from the federal government for a grant," said Gevins, "and about sixty cents of it would get wasted by the university.

It was just very inefficient, you know? The accounting was all wrong, the secretaries couldn't read and write, the floors were dirty, the windows weren't washed. . . . Once, I lined up a great deal on a computer, a once-in-a-lifetime deal, and they wouldn't let me buy it immediately. It took six months to get the paperwork approved. By that time the computer was gone."

Gevins's complaints about the academic bureaucracy are undoubtedly echoed in nearly every large college and university. His response, however, was far from the typical one. In 1981 he took the lab out of the University of California at San Francisco and established it as an independent entity. "We set it up as a nonprofit research institute," explained Gevins, "completely separated from the university. We have our own human-subjects research board; we have our own accounting department—the government auditors come directly to me. It was a risky thing to do back then, because who ever heard of a nonprofit, human-brain-wave research laboratory?

"But, you know, it worked out really well."

Gevins's initial monetary support came from an Air Force research laboratory; and soon he was pulling in grants from the Office of Naval Research, the National Institutes of Health, and the National Science Foundation. Like other institutions that seek federal grant money for scientific work, Gevins's EEG Systems Lab must compete. He explained, "I write a grant, it goes to peer review, and lots of times they're not funded. So we support ourselves just by writing grants, by competing with other scientists and universities."

Gevins and his team continue to get the good grants, and not only because they're good grant writers. They do good scientific work—work that is elucidating the connections between the brain and the body. Work that, as we'll see later, is also shedding light on the connection between the brain and the mind.

THE BRAIN AND THE BODY

That the brain controls the body, of course, is a given. It's one of those "everyone knows" kinds of things. Yet we continue to gain fascinating insights into just *how* the brain controls the body, in part with the imaging tools developed by Alan Gevins and others.

Some areas in the cerebral cortex, that extensive network of tightly packed and interconnected network of neurons that surrounds the forebrain, have hundreds of millions of neurons with connections leading deep into the brain. These connections reach all the way down to the brain stem, the part of the brain sitting just above the spinal cord. There these neural "wires" from the cerebral cortex link up with motor neurons. These are the nerve cells that carry signals to and from the muscles in our body.

In fact, so vital are the connections to the body's muscles that the brain uses at least seven different subsystems to control the body's motor activities. Automatic reflex pathways in the spine pull our hands away if we touch a hot stove or cause us to jump reflexively at a sudden alarming noise. A subsystem of neurons in the brain stem helps us keep our balance as we walk. Another brainstem subsystem responds to commands from the cerebral cortex by sending "act" or "don't act" signals to muscles that control posture. A neural pathway coming out of the area of the brain known as the midbrain also helps coordinate our body's posture, with signals coming from our eyes and ears.

The cerebellum—located at the base of the brain and looking like a pleated, spherical Chinese fan—helps to control the direction, rate, force, and steadiness of our conscious, intentional movements. When I consciously stretch my hand out and lift a cup of coffee to my lips, this subsystem goes into action. It compares the movement actually taking place with the intended movement and signals the correct areas in the brain needed to make the necessary adjustments.

Two other neural pathways link the cerebral cortex directly to the brain stem and spinal cord. They help control the precise movements we make when we are learning some physical activity. When my father was learning the violin in high school, for example, these areas in his brain's cerebral cortex helped control his hands and fingers. Finally, another neural pathway makes sure our muscles move smoothly as we walk, run, and come to a halt and helps control the unconscious movements we make when we are eating or walking.

Nearly all the nerve impulses that command specific muscular actions originate in the brain's motor cortex. The motor cortex stretches across the top of the brain from left to right, along a path that's just in front of our ears. Different areas of the motor cortex control the movements of specific muscles in the body. From our lips to our toes, each set of muscles has a corresponding region in the motor cortex.

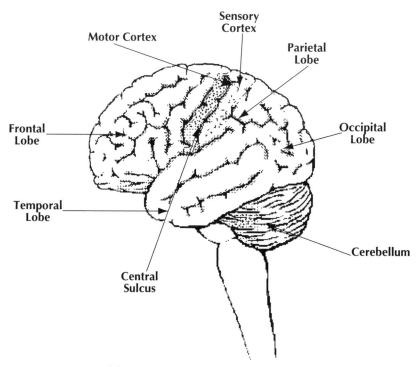

Motor Cortex

Sensory Cortex

Parietal Lobe

Frontal Lobe

Occipital Lobe

Temporal Lobe

Cerebellum

Central Sulcus

FIG. 5.1.   Some of the major parts of the brain's motor and sensory system.

The rearmost part of the motor cortex is called the somatosensory cortex. It handles information coming from various sensory receptors in the body. Many of the regions in the somatosensory cortex correspond directly to the same areas in the rest of the motor cortex. We'll get a closer look at the somatosensory cortex later on.

Some researchers have placed electrodes in patients' brains (with their permission) to record the activity of individual neurons. These experiments are usually done with subjects about to undergo brain surgery, usually to control epileptic seizures. These recordings reveal that electrical activity in specific regions of the motor-cortex regions is directly associated with movements of different limbs. Stimulate one specific region in the motor cortex and your left thumb will twitch. Stimulate another region and one of your calf muscles trembles. Another region and your right eyelid blinks.

Thousands of these kinds of experiments have been carried out over the last sixty years or so. The result is a detailed, functional map of this small but highly important region of the brain. This map* shows an orderly distribution of areas in the motor cortex that correspond to all the muscles of the leg, trunk, arm, and face.

One fascinating aspect of this map is how it shows the relative importance to the brain of certain muscles. The muscles in our fingers, lips, and tongue, for example, must carry out very precise and delicate movements. Sure enough, the areas in the motor cortex that control these muscles are disproportionately large. The muscles in our backs do not have to carry out such precise motions. Their regions in the motor cortex are relatively smaller.

The command-and-control relationship between the body and the brain is complex (see Fig. 5.2). Many of the areas of the brain involved in muscle control lie deep in the brain; the thalamus and basal ganglia are just two such regions. The cerebellum and brain stem, as we saw a little earlier, are at the base of the brain, close to the top of the spinal cord.

Commands from the brain can follow a complex set of pathways to eventually reach the skeletal muscles. In turn, information from various sensors in and around the muscles flows back to the brain in a continual feedback loop. This information lets the various parts of the motor cortex know what the body's muscles and bones are doing and whether or not they're doing what they've been told to do.

WILDER PENFIELD AND THE MOTOR CORTEX

During the first several decades of the twentieth century, brain researchers and doctors began to develop methods for probing the living brains of human patients. These probes involved the electrical stimulation of the exposed brains of otherwise conscious patients during neurosurgery. One of the pioneers in this kind of brain research was the American-Canadian neurosurgeon Wilder Penfield.

Penfield was born in Spokane, Washington, in 1891 and graduated from Princeton in 1913. He went on to become a Rhodes Scholar at Oxford in Great Britain. While there, he worked under the great British neurosurgeon Sir Charles Sherrington and developed his lifelong fasci-

*Called the motor homunculus because it is often represented by an exaggerated drawing of a human figure.

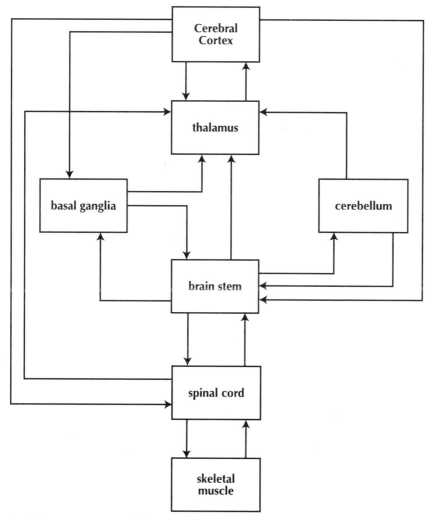

FIG 5.2   Major parts of the motor system in vertebrates. This schematic diagram shows the major connections among the primary components of the motor system in vertebrate animals. The arrows show the main neural connections between the different parts of the system.

nation with the brain. Penfield returned to the United States and in 1918 received his medical degree from Johns Hopkins University in Baltimore. In 1921, after a year interning in Boston and two years back at Oxford, Penfield began a neurosurgery practice in New York City.

Seven years later, he accepted an appointment as professor of neurology and neurosurgery at McGill University in Montreal, Canada. Eventually, he became a naturalized Canadian citizen.

Starting in the late 1920s and continuing through the 1950s, Penfield carried out some pioneering work on mapping the human brain. His brain-mapping efforts grew out of his work curing people suffering from focal epilepsy. Focal epilepsy is caused by tiny scars in certain parts of the brain. People suffering from focal epileptic seizures often experience hallucinations, overwhelming feelings of elation, depression or fear, foul odors, and muscle spasms. Penfield's surgical techniques for removing the scar tissue that was causing the seizures gave him an opportunity to do some more experimental work. Part of his technique involved stimulating the exposed cerebral cortex with microelectrodes. This technique allowed him to reduce the damage to the brain from the surgery itself. He soon discovered that touching parts of the exposed cerebral cortex in his conscious patients with the microelectrodes had remarkable side effects.

Some of the brain's blood vessels have pain sensors, but the nerves in the brain itself do not. Other nerves in the body do have pain sensors, at least in the glial sheaths surrounding them. But our brains have evolved without internal pain sensors connected to its own neurons. Perhaps the brain can't be bothered with feeling pain in itself but must concentrate on processing sensory input from the body, including pain signals.

Because the brain itself feels no pain, patients undergoing some kinds of brain surgery can be conscious during the entire process. A local anesthetic is used when the top of the skull is removed, stopping any pain signals that would come from the brain's blood vessels. But the person can remain completely conscious and aware while his or her brain is operated on.

First, Penfield would get permission from the patient for his experiment. Then, either before or after the actual neurosurgery, he would stimulate areas of the person's cerebral cortex with tiny electrical impulses delivered through a needle. The patient would suddenly respond, entirely involuntarily, to the electrical stimulation. When the temporal lobes were stimulated, the person might experience powerful recollections of past experiences, such as the smell of apple pie baking in mother's oven or a sudden visual memory of some kind.

When Penfield stimulated parts of the motor-cortex strip across the top of the brain, different parts of the patient's body would twitch or otherwise move. After years of work, Penfield was able to produce his "motor homunculus" map of the motor cortex. (Homunculus is a Latin word that means "little man.") The motor-homunculus map pinpoints areas in the motor cortex controlling different parts of the body. It also shows the relative sensitivity of some body parts and the importance of their movement to our daily lives. For example, a larger part of the motor cortex is devoted to the control of the hands and fingers than to the control of the muscles in the back. The homunculus map therefore has exaggerated hands and fingers, while the back is tiny.

During the course of this experimental mapping of the brain, Penfield discovered a previously unknown part of the motor cortex. Penfield named this patch of neural tissue, located along the top of the brain's cerebral cortex, the supplementary motor area, or SMA. Neuroscientists are only now beginning to uncover some of its complex activities. At the time of his death, however, Penfield had come up with his own, somewhat unorthodox, idea of the SMA's role. Unlike most other neurosurgeons, Penfield was a "dualist." He believed that the mind was an entity somehow separate from, but connected to, the brain. It had some kind of nonphysical reality, he thought. And he believed that the SMA was the place where the mind connected to—or "interfaced," as computer geeks would say today—with the brain.

Penfield created his motor-cortex map using electrocortical stimulation of the brain. This is an invasive procedure, of course. The researcher is usually a neurosurgeon who has lifted off the top of the patient's skull and is working on the naked, exposed brain. But at the time Penfield was working, it was the most advanced brain-imaging technology available.

KEN GRIFFEY JR. AND THE MOTOR CORTEX

In 1992 my former wife, Marie Celestre, died suddenly at age forty-five of a cerebral hemorrhage. A blood vessel at the back of her brain suddenly ruptured. In less than a second she was completely unconscious. Probably within a minute or two, all of her higher brain functions had stopped for good. Yet she continued breathing normally for another half an hour. Her death was sudden, tragic, seemingly meaningless—though, in truth, she had lived a vibrant and very meaningful life, one that indelibly touched thousands of other people and left them better human beings.

One remarkable medical fact stands out from this sad event. The most primitive parts of the brain can control muscle movements in the body even when the rest of the brain is dead. As long as certain regions of the brain stem and parts of the forebrain remain undamaged, a human body will continue to live, breathe, and even digest food. The *person* is gone; self-awareness, consciousness of the outside world, language, laughter, infectious smile, complex thought, are gone. But the basic bodily functions continue.

Of course, most of us for most of our lives have fairly intact and functioning brains. Many muscle movements do lie beyond our conscious control. We do not deliberately choose to pull our hand back from a hot stove, and most of the time we do not consciously order our eyelids to blink. But many other body movements we either consciously make or had to learn.

The basic muscle movements for walking, for example, seem to be programmed into the brain stem and spinal cord. But walking itself is something we must *learn* to do. Walking and running involve a complex set of muscle movements, coordinated with our senses of sight and balance. Watching an infant learning to walk, as my family watched my brother Tim nearly forty years ago, is proof that this is a learned skill, one that improves with practice. The child that is barely toddling at eighteen months will be trotting along next to Mom in the shopping mall by the time he is four. Those thirty months of practice make all the difference. And by that time, walking and running are pretty much nonconscious. The child does not have to consciously make the effort to move his or her legs properly or work to keep in balance. It's all learned now and happens without thinking about it.

Or consider the act of catching a fly ball in a baseball game. Randy "the Big Unit" Johnson fires a blazing fast ball. Cecil Fielder swings from the ankles; the ball leaves his bat with a crack and streaks out toward the deep recesses of Yankee Stadium. Ken Griffey Jr. watches for just an instant and then turns and runs like hell for the fences. The crowd rises to its feet, screaming with excitement. Griffey doesn't even slow down. At the last instant, he looks up and back over his shoulder, lifts his gloved hand, and wham! hits the padded outfield fence and slides to the dirt of the warning track. Up he leaps, ball in glove. Despite its partisan leanings, the crowd screams again, this time with respectful approval.

How on earth did he do it? Neuroscientists are beginning to know.

We already have a good idea of the general neurological picture of catching a fly ball. The moment the ball leaps from the bat into the sky,

Griffey's eyes have spotted it and started following its trajectory. His brain instantly begins computing its path through space. Millions of neural instructions flash instant by instant to hundreds of different muscles in his body. They tell those muscles how to run, where to run, how to hold his body in a dynamic balance that will increase his speed and with exactly the right degree of relaxation and tension from moment to moment. Meanwhile, his brain continues to compute the ball's trajectory and to predict where it will be at a given moment in time.

Griffey's running hell-bent for leather toward the outfield fence. His eyes send that information to the brain's visual system and thence to other neural networks. Those networks are computing the rapidly closing distance to the fence, how long it will be before he gets there, and when the *ball* will appear. At the last instant, he looks up and back over his shoulder. He spots the ball for an instant. In that moment, his brain receives the data from his visual cortex (at the back of the brain), makes final "midcourse corrections," and orders the arm up and out to precisely the correct spot in space where the ball should be at that instant. It is. He catches it. He hits the wall. His brain has already ordered his muscles to relax! as he hits. Oh. But don't relax the muscles in the hand with the glove and the ball.

Was all of this unconscious? Much of it was. But at some point Griffey learned how to run fast, catch well, and do some incredible midair acrobatics. And each time he runs for the ball, he *chooses* to do so.

ALMOST EVERY movement we make, conscious or unconscious, begins with the firing of a neuron or group of neurons in our brains. Many brain researchers think the initial spark, the nascent "will to move," is ignited in the motor cortex at the top of the brain. One demonstration of how that may happen has come from the work of Apostolos Georgopoulos and his colleagues.

Georgopoulos has his laboratories at the University of Minnesota and the Minneapolis Veteran's Administration Medical Center. For more than fifteen years he has conducted a series of experiments with monkeys. He eavesdrops on the activities of their brains as they carry out simple motor tasks, such as pushing a lever against resistance.

He has not used the new imaging technologies for this work, but has relied on the tried-and-true technology of individual embedded electrodes. This is not the kind of experiment that one can carry out on humans. Even if you or I gave Georgopoulos permission to do so, his local human-subjects board would probably not allow it. But this is an accepted technique with experimental animals, such as monkeys and mice. For the record, the animals do not feel any pain from these experiments. They're anesthetized when the electrodes are implanted, and there is no evidence that they find them painful or bothersome afterward. The electrodes are, in fact, sensors that can directly read the electrical activity of different neuron clusters. Some electrodes have probes so thin, in fact, that they can directly detect the electrical activity of individual neurons.

Georgopoulos inserts the electrodes into specific regions in the monkey's motor cortex. He focuses on the few hundred or so that control arm movements in the monkeys being studied. Georgopoulos's goal, he has said, is to "intercept the messages of the cells . . . as they communicate with other cells."

He and other researchers expected to find that different neurons in that area of the motor cortex were responsible for different directions of arm movement. Should the monkey move its arm to the left, one neuron would fire. Movement to the right would be signaled by a different neuron. It made a certain amount of sense. As we saw earlier, the detailed map of the human motor cortex does show how specific parts of the brain control specific muscles in the body.

That's not quite what Georgopoulos found. The neurons in the motor cortex do seem to have a "preferred direction," as he has put it, but their activities are considerably more complex than assumed. Any given neuron appears to be involved in *all* muscle movements in the arm. The catch is that this involvement lessens as the movement differs more and more from the one that the neuron "prefers." Thus, a particular neuron in Ken Griffey's motor cortex may send commands to a particular muscle or muscles to move his arm to the right. That same neuron will also be involved in sending signals to move the arm to the right and slightly upward, but its involvement is not as great as in the first situation. It is even less involved in sending commands to those particular muscles to move straight up. This is also the case with all the other neurons in the particular region of the motor cortex controlling Ken Griffey's catching arm.

In other words, according to Georgopoulos, the individual nerve cells continually "vote" for their preferred direction, but their votes are weighted. The strength of their votes depends on how close that particular direction is to the direction that Griffey *wants* to move his arm. It's as if a hundred people got together in a smoke-filled room somewhere to pick the next president of the United States. Let's say that there are three candidates: a liberal, a conservative, and a middle-of-the-road moderate. Each person gets a vote, each person has a preferred candidate, and each can vote for any of the three candidates.

The catch is, the votes are weighted by how close the candidate's political philosophy is to the candidate *I* want to win.

Suppose I want the liberal candidate to be president. If you vote for him, your vote is equal to one full vote. If you vote for the moderate, your vote is equal to half of a vote. And if your preferred candidate is the conservative, your vote is equal to just one-fourth of a full vote. The same setup exists for the other ninety-nine people in this room. The outcome of the election is determined by adding all the votes.

A somewhat similar process seems to take place in the area at the top of the brain that governs our body's movements, the motor cortex. The individual neurons in any particular region vote for their preferred direction, and each vote has a strength directly proportional to how close that direction is to the direction that Griffey wants to move his arm. The votes sum up, and the arm moves. He catches the ball, and the evening sportscasts have another "Griffey highlight" for the viewers.

While most of Georgopoulos's work has been done with invasive microelectrodes, he has also put the power of the computer to work for him. He and his colleagues have developed a nifty computer program that displays in vivid, graphic form just how this democratic process occurs. The program represents the vote of each neuron as a vector, which is basically a kind of mathematical arrow. Each vector, or arrow, points in the preferred direction of that particular neuron. The length of each arrow corresponds directly to the strength of that neuron's vote, that is, its signal or firing rate. The computer program then adds up all the vectors to produce what Georgopoulos and his colleagues call the "population vector."

So what exactly is happening in the monkey's brain as it pushes that lever? Georgopoulos and his team created an experimental setup to which the monkey would respond. A circular screen, like a clock face, had a handle at its center and a light that could flash at any location on its perimeter. The monkey's job was to grab the handle when the light flashed and move it toward an unlit point ninety degrees away from the light, in a counterclockwise direction. This is not a task that monkeys instinctively know. They have to learn it. What's more, they have to *think* about it; that is, they must plan it out in advance when they perceive the stimulus.

As the monkeys in Georgopoulos's experiments carried out their tasks, the electrodes in their motor cortexes detected the activity of the neurons. That information then went into a computer, where the "voter program" stored it, analyzed it, and created computer images of the neuronal activity.

The images created by the computer are, essentially, images of the monkeys' thought processes as they carried out their motor tasks. The population vector—that mathematical arrow that was the sum of all the arrows representing the direction and strength of each neuron's vote—would rotate from the direction of the stimulus to the required angle. If the stimulus was at the twelve o'clock position, for example, the population vector's graphic image would start rotating counterclockwise from that position. Millisecond by millisecond, the neurons in the motor cortex would change their firing rates. In about 130 milliseconds—less than one-seventh of a second—the arrow would sweep backwards to the nine o'clock position. About three hundredths of a second *later*, on the average, the monkey's arm would begin to move the lever to the correct location.

A note of caution here: The population vector that is being painted onto the computer screens in Georgopoulos's laboratory is not "real." It is a mathematical construct.° What appears on the computer monitor, or in hard-copy illustrations created by the program, does not literally exist in the monkey's brain. It is a mathematical representation of what appears *to be going on in the monkey's brain* as it prepares to carry out a set of muscle movements in one arm.

Moreover, it's important to remember that the monkey probably doesn't "see" its arm move in its "mind's eye" any more than Ken Griffey Jr. sees his arm move in *his* mind's eye as he reaches for that fly ball. Instead, Georgopoulos has said, this is "a motor rehearsal, a practicing of movement."

And, finally, let's remember that no one has stuck microelectrodes in Ken Griffey's head. No one has actually measured his motor neurons' firing rates as he catches that ball. We assume that what's happening in the monkey's motor cortex happens in ours. But that's a pretty safe assumption. We are evolutionary cousins to our primate companions on this planet. Our distant ancestors are the same, our genetic codes are practically identical. For all we know, a few random twists of fate a few million years ago could easily have put us in the shoes of Cousin Rhesus and him in ours.

°Which means, of course, that it's real for mathematicians, who, for the most part, are convinced that mathematical reality is the *only* reality.

MRI AND HANDEDNESS

Most of Georgopoulos's work has been with monkeys and microelectrodes, but he has recently been involved in an exploration of the motor cortex using MRI. One of the most exciting of the new imaging technologies in use today, MRI in its new versions, can provide researchers with images of the living brain in near-real-time action. This souped-up version of MRI is called functional MRI, or fMRI. Instead of taking "exposures" of brain activity over several minutes, researchers can now take "snapshots" of the brain in action that take only a second or two. A normal photograph taken with an exposure time of a minute will be very blurred. Only the largest details will be visible. A photo with an exposure time of a second or less will show much more detail. It's much the same with fMRI. Brain researchers can use this new imaging method to see much greater detail in how different parts of the brain function from moment to moment.

MRI had moved from the physics labs to the medical clinics in the late 1970s and early 1980s. That's when a researcher named Paul Lauterbur, at the University of Illinois, discovered how to use NMR (nuclear magnetic resonance) to create noninvasive body images by magnetically jiggling the protons inside atoms. In 1990, Seiji Ogawa and his associates at the AT&T Bell Labs conjured up fMRI. His new twist on this technology made it the hottest technology in medical imaging.

When neurons work hard, firing quickly and repeatedly, they gobble up larger than normal amounts of glucose, the sugar compound that is the brain's major source of food. However, researchers, using positron emission tomography, or PET scans, had already discovered a curious aspect to the life of neurons. Active brain areas consume more glucose but don't use additional oxygen. For reasons still unknown, brain neurons that are working hard and firing frequently behave a lot like the leg muscles of a sprinter. Those muscles also use up glucose rapidly but do not use correspondingly more oxygen. Run too fast, too long, too hard, and your leg muscles start to cramp, in part as a result of oxygen starvation.

In the same way, the blood vessels feeding the brain its glucose are delivering lots of oxygen to the active areas. But it's oxygen that doesn't get used. This means that the small veins carrying blood away from active brain areas have a high concentration of oxygen in them. It's a traffic jam of oxygen on the way out of the brain.

Back in 1935 the famous biochemist Linus Pauling made an interesting discovery about oxygen in the blood. A molecule called hemoglobin is the "truck" that carries oxygen.* Pauling discovered that the amount of oxygen in the hemoglobin will affect hemoglobin's magnetic properties. Fifty-five years later, Ogawa and his associates showed that MRI could detect these small magnetic fluctuations in blood. Within eighteen months several research teams had developed ways to use MRI to detect changes in blood-oxygen levels in the brain caused by specific brain functions. This is why the technique is called *functional* MRI, or fMRI.

fMRI has several advantages over computerized tomography (CT) and PET scanning. First, fMRI provides both functional and anatomic information about the brain. Also, the signal it detects comes directly from the changes in the brain tissue. Unlike PET, nothing radioactive need be injected beforehand into the patient to detect a signal. The spatial resolution of fMRI is also better than that of PET. That is, fMRI can detect structures as small as 1–2 millimeters—much smaller than the smallest structure PET can image. Finally, certain versions of fMRI can also monitor these functional changes in blood flow in the brain in near-real time. And as we've just seen, that means clearer images with less "blurring," sharper images of the brain in action from instant to instant.

The only drawbacks to fMRI currently known are the same ones known for earlier versions of the technique. It is extremely loud; MRI uses extremely powerful magnets whose mechanical parts bang disturbingly loud each time the magnetic field is triggered. So loud are MRI machines that people being imaged have to wear earplugs. Some patients suffer claustrophobia from the close quarters in which they must lie inside some machines.

Some scientists and others have also worried about possible deleterious side effects from the strong magnetic fields used. However, every test done so far on this aspect of MRI has shown no harmful effects. The worst that happens is a feeling of dizziness that can take place in a room filled with an MRI imager's extremely powerful magnetic field. The magnetic field is so strong, hundreds to thousands of time stronger than the earth's magnetic field, that it can disrupt the organs in the inner ear that control our sense of balance.

The remarkable abilities of fMRI made it an ideal imaging technique for a series of experiments carried out in 1993 by Georgopoulos and several colleagues. They were interested in the connection between the motor cortex, brain asymmetry, and handedness.

---

*It also gives blood its red color.

Most of us are familiar with handedness. A good 90 percent of the general population is right-handed. No other species on earth appears to have this propensity. A fifty-fifty distribution of handedness prevails in every other species studied, including our primate cousins. Nor does genetics seem to play a role in handedness. About 85 percent of all left-handed children (like myself) have two right-handed parents.

What many people do not know is that, as we've noted earlier, the brain itself has a certain handedness. This is scientifically referred to as "hemispheric asymmetry." For example, in most people the speech centers of the brain are located in the cerebral cortex's left hemisphere. The parts of the brain that process spatial tasks and the spatial distribution of attention are located in the right cerebral hemisphere. Most of us are "left-brained" for language and "right-brained" for stacking boxes one on top of the other.*

This asymmetry also extends to the consequences of damage to the motor cortex. Damage to the left hemisphere's part of the motor cortex usually has a more pronounced effect on a person's body than does damage to the motor cortex in the right hemisphere. Damage to a particular area of the right motor cortex will paralyze the person's left hand and vice-versa. At the same time, the motor function of the "ipsilateral" hand—the hand on the same side of the body as the affected cerebral hemisphere—can also be affected by such a stroke.

Strangely enough, the severity of the paralysis in this "isplateral" or same-side hand depends on the hemisphere in which the damage occurred. If the motor cortex in the left hemisphere is damaged by a stroke or other injury, the person's left hand will often suffer some dysfunction. But if the damage is to the right side of the motor cortex, the person's right hand is almost always unaffected.

A few researchers have studied this curious phenomenon, but none of them paid attention to the handedness of the people they studied. Georgopoulos decided to look into this and to begin at the beginning. The beginning was simple: First, determine if there's a difference between the activation of the right and left sides of the motor cortex. And second, uncover what relationship, if any, might exist between a person's handedness and this kind of motor-cortex activation.

---

*I hesitate to use "left-brain" and "right-brain," but they are the best phrases possible in this case. Far too much nonsense has been published about the left brain versus the right brain. In fact, we each have *one* brain with two hemispheres.

Georgopoulos's study included fifteen healthy people with an average age of about thirty-one years. Ten were right-handed (five women and five men). The others, four men and a woman, were left-handed. Each took a turn snuggling into the barrel of an MRI machine. As they lay there, they were to touch their thumb to the tips of each of the other four fingers in turn. The MRI machine created images of their brains before, during, and after they carried out these simple movements. Each person repeated this task in random order with each hand, thus activating each side of their motor cortex.

What the researchers found was a clear asymmetry, or "handedness," in the way the two sides of the motor cortex work in humans. This is particularly pronounced in the right-handed people studied. For example, the right motor cortex was activated mostly during opposite-side finger movements by both right-handers and left-handers. But the left motor cortex often went into action not only during same-side finger movements by left-handers but even more so when it was *right-handers* making the same-side finger movements.

Georgopoulos believes that the left motor cortex's notable involvement in these ipsilateral, or same-side, finger movements could help explain the fact that damage to the left—but not the right—motor cortex causes significant paralysis in a person's hand on the same side of the body. It happens that about 10–15 percent of the nerve fibers coming out of these areas of the motor cortex do *not* cross to the other side of the brain. Georgopoulos thinks there's a connection between that fact and the asymmetry the MRI scans discovered.

The work by Georgopoulos and his colleagues with monkeys is just one good example of how research on the motor cortex is moving into new territory even without the benefit of the new imaging technologies. And his study of the human motor cortex with MRI shows how these new imaging machines are also being used to probe the mysteries of the brain and its connection to our muscles.

Meanwhile, more than two thousand miles to the west of Georgopoulos's lab in Minneapolis, Alan Gevins is using his new version of an old imaging technology to do the same thing.

EEG AND BRAIN MAPS

About twenty-five people work with Gevins at the EEG Systems Laboratory. According to Gevins, it's a completely interdisciplinary shop that includes Ph.D.s and engineers. The laboratory works in fields that range from electrical engineering and mechanical engineering to computer science and mathematics, from neurocognitive physiology and neuroscience to cognitive psychology. "All the pieces we need are here in the lab," Gevins explained. "We can design circuits for amplifiers, which we do. We write all our own software. We have about five people who do nothing but program. We do the experiments and even write the philosophical treatises. It's a vertically integrated operation, if you will."

What Gevins and his team have done is to take the old-fashioned EEG and learn how to extract a lot more information from it. This has been possible in part because Gevins himself has a background in both engineering and neuroscience and because the laboratory has a long history of focusing exclusively on the EEG as a brain-mapping tool. By putting together a team of talented people, Gevins is actualizing his dream of measuring the brain's activities in real time, using a souped-up version of an imaging technology that's well over seventy years old. Just as newer is not necessarily better, older is not necessarily worse.

"Measuring brain waves has several advantages over some of the other methods that you will hear about," said Gevins, "and I think that there are some disadvantages, too.

"PET scanning, positron emission tomography, I think was a method of the eighties. Functional MRI is the method of the nineties. What these two imaging technologies give is complete precision in three dimensions about the metabolic activity throughout the brain. That's their advantage.

"What they *lack*," added Gevins, "is the time resolution to resolve something that lasts just a few milliseconds. PET resolves about sixty seconds. Functional MRI seems to resolve about two seconds, although I'm sure they'll figure out how to make it faster. So their time resolution is a little smeared. That's important if you're interested in thinking in the brain. Thinking is very fast. If you have a shutter that is wide open as a race car goes by, when you take a look at the picture, it's blurred. With PET and MRI, researchers must go through a lot of juggling to try to see some kind of image of thought. And they make up controls and subtract one thing from the other; there's a lot of hope and prayer in what they do."

On the other hand, added Gevins, his souped-up EEG has a temporal resolution that is measured in fractions of a second. Another advantage to his technique is that it is very portable. Said Gevins, "You can record [brain waves during] conversations in a room, like this. We recorded a race car driver a couple of months ago. We did it *while* he was driving. We've recorded people flying airplanes, people operating radar units, most anything."

"This technology provides us the only way of looking at the brain in the real world; there's no other method that can go out of the laboratory. You can't take a PET scanner with you!" he said, laughing. "Perhaps you have heard of MEG, magnetoelectroencephalograms." MEG is a method for measuring the magnetic fields generated by the brain's electrical activity. "That also can't go out of the laboratory; that's a very, very delicate measurement."

Unlike PET, MRI, MEG, and other current imaging technologies, EEG is cheap. The amplifiers used in the machine cost Gevins a few dollars in parts for each channel. "It's all software and computing," said Gevins. "It's a signal-processing problem."

But EEG has its disadvantages as well, For one thing, it's not a true three-dimensional imaging method. Gevins cannot use EEG to image some particular activity anywhere in the brain. He can, under special conditions, measure activity in the brain stem. And he can measure activity in the superficial cortex fairly easily, particularly in areas of the temporal, parietal, and prefrontal cortexes.

"I understand the limitations of this method. It is very good at seeing activity in the superficial exposed cortex, very good for that. It's not a very good modality if I was trying to perform neurosurgery to determine what area of the brain to take out." PET and functional MRI (fMRI) are much better imaging methods for that kind of task, said Gevins, even though they also have some limitations. "You can't record someone having a seizure on an MRI scanner, and yet you need to record the actual seizure itself to determine where it's coming from. EEG gives you signals of the action of hundreds of millions of neurons at a time. It's looking at the *input* to the *output* cells of the cortex."

The traditional EEG technology has had two weaknesses. First, most doctors or researchers traditionally use a set of nineteen or twenty-one electrodes for most EEG recordings. The electrodes are part of a special cap that fits over the head and which places the electrodes in specific locations on the skull. The distance between each electrode in this arrangement is about 7 centimeters, or about 2.75 inches.

Researchers who work with computer images often measure an image's dimensions in *pixels*, which is short for "picture elements." Each pixel has a color value or shade-of-gray value that's stored in the computer in bytes and then reproduced on the screen. A pixel that represents an area of the actual object that is black, for example, will have a byte value of 0. A pixel that is completely white may have a byte value of 254. An image with a lot of pixels has more detail to it than an image with fewer pixels. That's because each pixel represents a particular real-life area of the object in the image.

One way to picture this is to examine the three images in Figure 5.3. Imagine that each is a computerized "picture" of some object taken from the same distance and with the same lighting. Each has the same physical dimensions of, say, 12 centimeters high by 16 centimeters wide, or 192 square centimeters. The first computer image consists of four pixels, two across and two high. Each pixel in this image has an effective size of 48 square centimeters. The second computerized image is an array of sixteen pixels, four across and four down. Each pixel in this image has an effective size of 12 square centimeters, a resolution that's four times that of the first image. Finally, the third illustration is a "computer image" with sixty-four pixels, eight across and eight down. Each pixel in this image has an effective size of 3 square centimeters, a resolution four times as good as the second image and sixteen times that of the first.

For computer images created with traditional EEGs using a network of nineteen electrodes, each pixel would have the effective size of 49 square centimeters. Gevins uses a specially constructed skull network of 124 electrodes. The result is a vast improvement in image resolution. Instead of the resolution being 49 square centimeters to a pixel, it's about 5 square centimeters per pixel.

The other problem with all traditional EEG images, said Gevins, is that the human skull acts as an out-of-focus lens. When the electrical impulses generated by hundreds of millions of neurons travel from the surface of the brain to the scalp, the skull warps and blurs them. The brain waves are thus "out of focus." Gevins and his people at the EEG Systems Laboratory spent about ten years developing a method to remove this blurring effect. They call their technique, not surprisingly, deblurring.

Deblurring is done with sophisticated computer software, and Gevins has published the details of the technique in various industry journals. "It's neat," he said. "The spatial detail we are able to see in the EEG is much better than it used to be."

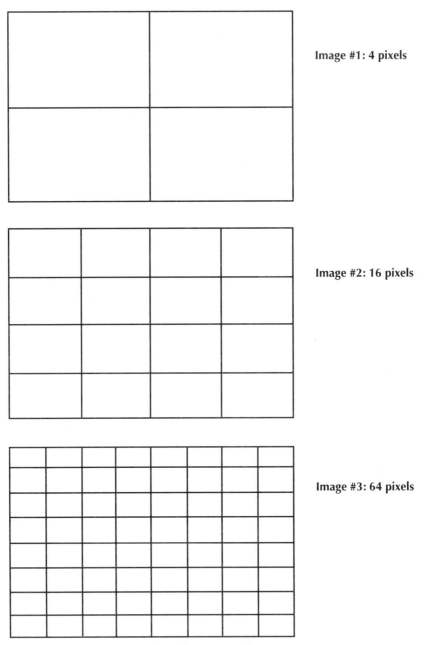

FIG. 5.3   Examples of pixels and image resolution.

What Gevins and EEG Systems have done is create a new kind of EEG imaging system. This new EEG imager can actually capture the thought *behind* a movement by creating images of brain-wave activity taken every four thousandths of a second. That's 250 times faster than the fastest fMRI imagers. These images show waves of electrical activity flowing like a lightning bolt across the brain.

In my meeting with him, Gevins relished talking about measuring brain-wave activity in football players, race-car drivers, and air-force test pilots. It was "neat," "fun." It was a totally new way of watching the brain at work—not in some sophisticated brain lab but "in the field," in the real world. Just as important, however, and perhaps even more important, are the insights that Gevins' new EEG technology is providing into how the brain responds to injuries and insults to the motor system.

One such dramatic finding had to do with a young woman from Wisconsin who had suffered a terrible stroke while giving birth. The stroke had damaged areas of the motor cortex in her brain's right hemisphere and thus paralyzed the left side of her body. The woman was able to recover the ability to move her left arm after considerable physical rehabilitation but still had some difficulty extending the arm to its full length. The woman's doctors were interested in finding out what had happened in her brain during her recovery from the stroke. They contacted Gevins and then flew the woman to San Francisco for a series of EEG imaging sessions.

What Gevins discovered flew in the face of a long-established "given" about the brain and lateralization. His highly detailed EEG images clearly showed that the woman's brain had moved control of the muscle movements extending her left arm from the damaged area in the right hemisphere's part of the motor cortex. Those muscles were now being commanded by a new spot in her brain's left hemisphere. At the same time, the normal area in the right side of the motor cortex continued to control the muscles that flexed her left arm.

These images revealed that the brain is a lot more "plastic" and flexible than anyone had previously thought. They also showed the motor cortex in action in a way that had never been seen before. Like the work being done by Georgopoulos and his team with humans and MRI scanners, Gevins's research has revealed the existence of "same-sided" brain control of the body's muscles. This one small area of brain research is, in fact, one of the hottest areas of neuroscience in this Decade of the Brain.

Alan Gevins and Apostolos Georgopoulos are not the only researchers using new and old imaging technologies to learn about the brain's motor cortex. For example, Stephen Lisberger of the University of California at San Francisco works with monkeys who wear special spectacles. The glasses change the monkeys' view of the world. Lisberger studies how their distorted vision of the world affects the firing of neurons in their motor cortexes as the monkeys try to follow a moving target with their eyes. At the National Institute of Neurological Disorders and Stroke, Alvaro Pascual-Leone works with healthy adult human volunteers who are learning to play the piano for the first time. He studies how the motor areas in their brains change as they learn this new skill.

These discoveries about the brain's motor cortex are fascinating in themselves—as examples of pure science for knowledge's sake. But as we'll see later on, these new revelations about the connections between the brain and the body have important practical implications. They will give us new insights into lifelong learning and into recovery from devastating brain injuries.

CHAPTER 6

THE BRAIN AND THE SENSES

IN 1986 I was finishing work on my second book, *Flyby: The Inter-planetary Odyssey of Voyager 2*. My editor asked me if I knew anyone who would write a short introduction for it. I suggested Isaac Asimov; my editor thought that sounded great, and so I called "the Good Doctor" to ask if he'd do it. Asimov answered the phone, and his voice sounded a bit muffled. In fact, he had a terrible cold. He asked a few questions and sounded somewhat dubious. As usual, he was busy writing several books at once, plus his next science column for *Fantasy & Science Fiction* magazine, and on and on. And then he changed the subject:

"Joel, I'm sorry I sound so awful. I've had this cold for days. But that's not what's really bad. You see, one of the consequences has been that I have completely lost my sense of taste. This is just terrible!" I laughed, since I knew well how much Isaac enjoyed a good meal; on a visit to New York a year earlier, we had had a delicious lunch at Tavern on the Green in Central Park.

"Ageusia," I replied.

"Ageusia?"

"Yes. It means loss of the sense of taste."

"*Ageusia!*" he repeated with delight. "Ageusia! What a wonderful word! Thank you very much!" At which point he agreed to write the introduction to *Flyby* as soon as I sent him a copy of the manuscript. "You know," he said as we finished our conversation, "this is turning out to be a good day. Not only did I get to talk with you, but *I learned a new word!*" I was flattered by the compliment; but I also knew how important learning a new word was to a man who knew so many.

THE MANY SENSES

Sensory reception is the mechanism that makes it possible for living beings to react to changes in their external and internal environments. All living creatures possess some sort of sensory mechanism. The single-celled creatures called prokaryotes (such as blue-green algae and lichens) are believed to be the descendants of the earliest complex creatures to appear on earth. Even these primitive organisms have senses. They all have some kind of "chemical sense," an ability to detect and respond to changes in the chemical composition of their outer environments. Many also have a primitive light sense. They can detect changes in light levels and react appropriately.

Plants do not have eyes, ears, or tongues. But they do have visual receptors that help them locate sources of light. Many of us have seen time-lapse motion pictures showing plants moving during the day to keep their leaves or blossoms pointed toward the sun. Plants also have a gravity sense, which helps them grow vertically. They have other senses that allow them to time the processes of germination and flowering with changes in temperature and length of daylight.

Most animals have the full complement of senses with which we are familiar. They depend on them to locate food, to avoid predators, and to monitor their environment. Highly acute senses can give an organism a decided survival advantage. And for us humans, our senses enliven our life experiences.

When my wife and I take a walk through one of the city parks near our home, we experience the world through our different senses. Our eyes capture the blue flash of a Steller's jay flying past. We smell the distinctive odor of pine needles from the trees around us. A light breeze blows through the trees, and we feel it brush our faces and arms. It's a cool breeze, and we feel momentarily chilled. We round the bend of the trail and see a blackberry bush. The berries look dark and ripe, and we try one. The bitter taste suggests they're not quite as ripe as we'd prefer. Down the trail and to the left is a small waterfall. The rushing sound of tumbling water alerts us before we see it.

All sensory receptors or sense cells have one common characteristic: Each is a specialized structure of a sensory nerve that is excited by a certain stimulus. The stimulus may be external or internal. Internal receptors allow the brain to constantly monitor the body's chemical and physical states. External receptors make it possible for a creature to continuously monitor the environment of the outer world. The brain uses this information to construct a continuously changing model of the external environment. And it does this in order to determine the creature's most appropriate response to changes in that environment.

The Greek philosopher Aristotle identified the five senses as sight, hearing, smell, taste, and touch. We now know of the existence of far more than the five classical senses. Special internal sensory receptors respond to mechanical or physical stimuli occurring inside the body. One such type of sensory receptor inside the ear and in the body's muscles and tendons maintains a sense of the body's position and movement in space. Stretch receptors in the muscles help the brain coordinate the expansion and contraction of muscle fibers, important in maintaining posture. Pain receptors are found throughout the body's tissues, both within the body as well as in the skin.

The sense we often refer to as touch is actually just one of several related senses, which include those dealing with gravity, muscle tone, pain, sound, touch, and vibration. An example: Every creature that moves freely on land needs to know from instant to instant that it is in some kind of dynamic balance and not falling over. This state of equilibrium is the relationship of the body to the pull of gravity. In humans, the brain gets this kind of information from special sensory hairs within the inner ear. These hairs are actually the receptors for the "vestibular sense," our sense of balance.

Another set of specialized sense receptors detect various kinds of vibrations passing through gases, liquids, or even solids. Only two major groups of animals actually possess a hearing or sound sense: insects and vertebrates, which include amphibians, birds, fish, and mammals. Sensory hairs and other specialized phonoreceptors are found in insects. All of the vertebrate animals that live in water have special sense receptors called lateral-line organs located in their outer skin. These descry faint water currents produced by other animals moving nearby. In vertebrates, two labyrinth-like structures next to the brain contain sensory endings that serve as sound receptors. Some species of fishes have acute hearing; others hear poorly. Bats, as most of us know, have an extraordinarily sophisticated mechanism for sound reception. They use a process called echolocation, bouncing sound waves off objects and listening to the reflected echoes. In humans the inner ear contains the sensory organs for hearing and equilibrium.

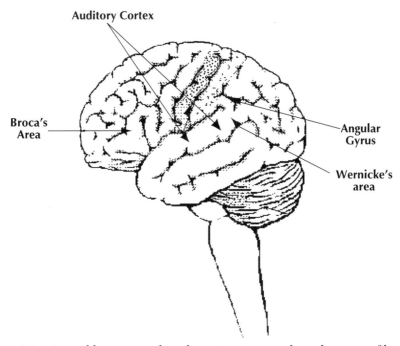

FIG. 6.1.   Several brain areas that play an important role in the sense of hearing include the auditory cortex, the angular gyrus, Broca's area, and Wernicke's area.

Still other receptors in the skin provide the brain with data about heat, cold, pressure, and noxious or painful stimuli. Snakes have small depressions or pits on their faces that contain temperature-sensitive sensory receptors. They use these receptors to detect the presence of nearby living creatures that might provide them with a meal. The antennae that many insects possess may provide them with thermal information.

Practically every living creature on the face of the earth possesses some sort of chemical sense. This surely must be the first and oldest of the senses. Even the most primitive creatures that ever existed would have needed to know about changes in the chemistry of their environment. Such changes would signal availability or absence of food, for example, or a change in oceanic salinity that might kill them. In humans and most other creatures, smell and taste are examples of chemical senses. The sensory cells that govern the chemical sense we call smell respond to chemicals that exist as gases or vapors. Olfactory (or smell) neurons in the nose provide the human brain with this kind of information. An organ in amphibians called Jacobsen's organ may well play a role in smell in that class of animal. Researchers have identified at least three different types of smell receptors in insects. Male moths, for example, sport big, bushy antennae that they use to detect special chemicals called pheromones released by female moths. Mice and other rodents, as well as many other mammals, appear to possess glands in the nasal area that detect these specialized chemical signals. Humans, too, may well respond to pheromones, but the evidence continues to be inconclusive about this.

In humans and most other vertebrates, the taste buds are the primary sensory cell for taste. These modified skin cells respond to chemicals in solution. Humans and most other vertebrates have taste cells in their mouths, on their tongues, and in their throats. Some species of fish have taste buds on the surface of their skin. In insects, the same receptors involved in smell appear to also play a role in taste. The four basic taste sensations in humans are sweet, sour, bitter, and salty. For that matter, most animals detect these four basic tastes. Many animals besides humans have a "sweet tooth," and the inborn abhorrence to bitter tastes appears to be nearly universal in animals. This isn't surprising; most poisonous substances have a bitter taste. So it makes sense that evolution would over time have genetically programmed into most creatures an aversion to the bitter taste.

Finally, most creatures have sensory organs or cells that are sensitive to various wavelengths of electromagnetic radiation—light. Light, in this case, is not just the visible light that we humans can detect with our eyes. Nor need these "photoreceptor" cells be structures as complex as the human eye. As noted earlier, most plants have cells that respond to light and darkness. Segmented worms have photoreceptor cells that simply detect different levels of light. The primitive eyespots found in many types of flatworms are photoreceptors. Arthropods, such as lobsters and various mollusks, have compound eyes that form images. So do many different types of insects. Bees are only one of many creatures that can see ultraviolet radiation (which causes sunburns). Still other creatures can, unlike humans, see infrared radiation—heat radiation.

In the last several years brain researchers have brought the full suite of imaging technologies to bear on the question of how the brain receives, stores, and interprets sensory information. Electro-encephalograms (EEG), CT (computerized tomography) scans, positron-emission tomography (PET), magnetic resonance imaging

(MRI), and other techniques are being used in labs around the world. All the senses are being studied with the new brain imagers. We can get a good idea of how brain researchers are using noninvasive imagery to study the senses by looking at some work being done with touch, hearing, and sight.

The first real breakthroughs in brain mapping using imaging technologies came with the invention and refinement of the PET scanner. One person who has been a major player in the development and use of PET is Marcus Raichle, of Washington University in St. Louis, Missouri.

THE PET PIONEER

Raichle started out professionally as a neurologist, working and studying at New York Hospital's Cornell Medical Center under Frederick Plum. "The interest in that laboratory was in brain circulation and metabolism," Raichle recalled during a long telephone conversation, "so I learned a good bit about how one goes about measuring that kind of stuff."

In the late 1960s the Vietnam War intervened, and Raichle spent two years in the air force. After his tour of duty, he moved to St. Louis, Missouri, in 1971. There he began working with physicists who wanted someone on their team who was interested in the brain and possibly had a background in that area. Raichle was soon looking into ways of using isotopes that emit positrons, the antimatter form of electrons, for medical purposes. Since the brain is so large, it was a relatively easy organ on which to try out various positron-emitting measuring techniques.

To Raichle, this work "sounded kind of nifty. And there were big cyclotrons involved and exotic isotopes, and we could make measurements that were impossible before." This was all taking place before PET scanning or MRI had even been invented. Raichle and the others were still able to build some rather elaborate testing equipment that allowed them to get some looks into the brain. Meanwhile, researchers in the Scandinavian countries had been carrying out measurements of blood flow in the brain using radioisotopes and learning how to relate them to specific brain functions. So Raichle knew it was possible to do those kinds of experiments on people.

He had been at Washington University for about two years when CT scanning was invented by Hounsfield and Cormack. Today Raichle leads a group of about thirty-five researchers. At that time, though, his research team consisted of himself, one other neurobiologist, and a bunch of physicists. "The first thing these guys wanted to do was to build a bigger and better CT scanner," he recalled with a chuckle. "They thought they could beat out Hounsfield, I guess. That whole episode is probably worth a chapter of its own in some book someday. But the upshot was that effort got derailed. So they were kind of looking around for what would be a logical project. Somebody decided, 'Well, geeze, we can reconstruct the density of the tissue by passing X rays through it. Maybe we could reconstruct the distribution of an isotope in the tissue if we looked at it in an emission sense.' And, of course, positron-emitting radionuclides were ideal for this.

"So they proceeded to tear apart these detecting devices that we had built because we didn't have anything else to build the scanner with." The Washington University group created its first tabletop device in 1973. Their first human PET image was created in April 1974. "Actually, it was an image of the brain," said Raichle. "It was obtained by injecting nitrous-13 ammonia as a radiotracer, which really didn't provide any functional information."

The team had already managed to get some information about brain function using its pre-PET imaging instruments, so that was the logical direction for them to go with their newly invented PET scanner. According to Raichle, the group still spent much of the 1970s developing the basic measurement techniques that would eventually become standard with PET. "We did fool around at times trying functional things," he said. But the more basic questions, such as measuring blood flow in the brain with PET, proved to be a lot more complicated than they had first anticipated.

At the same time, the machines themselves were undergoing considerable changes and improvements. "The first one, we called PET 3," Raichle said. "Then there was a PET 4, which had a lot of problems, and a PET 5, which coughed and burped. Finally, in 1980 we built PET 6, and for the next thirteen years we were able to produce some landmark stuff, I think, in terms of functional brain imaging."

Like a baby who crawls before it walks and walks before it runs, Raichle and his team started simple, "like moving the hands" and seeing what part of the brain "lit up" in the computer-created images. "A lot of that work was focused on how to go about studying these kind of things, on the kinds of techniques related to the image averaging, tracking techniques, and so forth," Raichle explained. "That all culminated in a 1988 paper we published in *Nature* on language and brain. From the vantage point of our group, I think that was kind of a landmark paper. Not so much that it revolutionized our way of thinking about language or anything. But it encapsulated probably fourteen years worth of work, everything from figuring out how to get the machine to work to learning out how to measure blood flow and stumbling and tripping through the whole business of tracking images and averaging images, and so forth.

"There were many dead ends along the way, but I think all of it came together in that paper." Raichle and his Washington University team have never looked back.

PET AND TOUCH

One of the areas in which the new brain-imaging technologies are making new discoveries is in the realm of the senses. A good example is the work being done by Raichle and one of his colleagues at Washington University, psychologist Wayne Drevets, studying the brain and the sense of touch.

Touch is the earliest of the human senses to develop. The various sensors that contribute to "touch" are already active by the time an embryo is seven weeks old. At that point, its ears and eyes have not yet developed. Newborn infants use their sense of touch to learn about their surroundings. Even after their senses of sight and hearing have matured, they will use touch to confirm those impressions. Watch as a young infant reaches out to touch her mother's face or smacks at the refrigerator as she is carried into the kitchen.

Numerous studies have confirmed that touch is the sense that creates the mother-child bond. Like the monkeys to whom we are cousins, as infants, we grab our mothers and hold on to them as much as possible. Conversely, most mothers will almost instinctively pick up their infants, hold them close, caress and fondle them. All that touching makes a difference. Children who are not well touched as infants almost always have greater difficulty learning, communicating, and forming healthy relationships than children who were given lots of hugs and loving touches.

As we saw earlier, the sense of touch is really one of several related senses. We actually have specific and separate senses for gravity (or equilibrium), heat, cold, pressure, muscle tone, and pain. Touch receptors in the skin are very sensitive. They respond not only to a whack on the arm with a large stick but also the gentle brush of a feather. In the latter case, the sequential activation of touch receptors by this gentle pressure may be interpreted by your brain as a "tickle."

One area of the brain that is involved in detecting and processing sensory information is the somatosensory cortex, a band in the brain's uppermost layer—the cerebral cortex—stretching from left to right across the top of the head. It lies just behind the motor cortex (which we explored in chapter 5). Behind the somatosensory cortex are the brain's parietal lobes and, behind that, the occipital lobe, at the back of the brain. As we saw in chapter 5, the somatosensory and motor cortexes have a close correspondence to specific parts of the body.

As with the motor cortex, different parts of the body are mapped to specific parts of the somatosensory cortex. This part of the brain responds to sensory inputs for heat, cold, pain, and the position of the body. The more sensitive a particular body part is to any of these inputs, the larger the area devoted to receiving and processing that information. In humans, for example, hands and fingers contain a large number of receptors for pressure, pain, heat, cold, and other related senses. The corresponding locations in the somatosensory cortex are much larger than the region devoted to, say, the big toe. Again, human lips are extremely sensitive to touch. Our backs are less so. This difference in sensitivity is also reflected in the somatosensory cortex.

Drevets and his colleagues were specifically interested in seeing what the brain does when it anticipates a particular stimulus. To do this, they used PET scans to measure the blood flow in the somatosensory cortexes of twenty-seven adult volunteers. First, each volunteer had PET scans taken of their brains while they lay in a quiet, relaxed, resting state. For these and the other PET scans, the subjects inhaled minuscule, harmless amounts of radioactively labeled oxygen. As we saw earlier, radioactive isotopes of oxygen are excellent tracers for PET scans, since the bloodstream carries the oxygen to the areas of the brain that are working hard.

For the first experiment, the researchers began by determining the "force thresholds" at which each volunteer would actually detect a gentle touch to the left or right big toe. Half of the volunteers had their left big toe stimulated with a tiny hairlike fiber; the other half had their right big toe brushed with the fiber. The point of determining the force thresholds was not for the benefit of the researchers. Rather, it was a way to get the volunteers to anticipate another touch to their toes.

Once they had determined the amount of force needed for the volunteers to feel a touch to their toes, the researchers and the subjects waited at least ten minutes. Then the volunteers inhaled the air laced with the radioactive isotopes of oxygen. The researchers reminded each volunteer which toe had been touched and asked them to be ready to count the number of times their toe was brushed. As the subjects anticipated the momentary touch to their left or right toes, the PET scanner recorded the activity in their brains. In fact, the researchers never did touch the volunteers' toes a second time. The whole point of the experiment was to see what happens in the brain when it is *anticipating* such a touch.

Then Drevets carried out a second experiment. This one involved painful but still harmless electrical shocks to the left or right index fingers of the volunteers. Once again, the researchers first determined how much electrical stimulation was needed for each subject to actually feel the shock. And as was the case in the first experiment, this was really not for the benefit of the researchers. It was meant to "prime" the volunteers to be ready for a shock they *knew* they would feel.

Again, the volunteers waited awhile before inhaling the radioactive oxygen; again, they anticipated a painful electrical shock at any moment to their left or right index fingers. Again, the PET scanner measured the activity taking place in their brains, particularly in the somatosensory cortex.

Finally, the researchers did a final experiment. This one must have been rather distressing to some of the volunteers. They deliberately focused on those people in the subject group who had some mild but nevertheless real animal fear of snakes or tarantulas. Would *you* like to have a tarantula suspended in a clear plastic cage 50 centimeters (about 3 feet) above your face? Or perhaps a small snake? That's what the researchers did. First the subjects spent three seconds looking at the animal. Then they closed their eyes, and about twenty seconds later, the animal was suspended above their faces. In each case there was no way that the tarantula or snake could escape and actually fall on them; the researchers assured the volunteers that this was so. It didn't matter, of course. We're talking about fear of tarantulas here. The PET scans took place while the subjects lay with their eyes closed, fearfully anticipating the "plop" of a snake or tarantula on their face at any moment.

Each PET scan represented an average of forty seconds of brain activity, a time frame fairly typical of PET scans. By subtracting the PET-scan readings made while the volunteers were resting from the ones recorded during anticipation, Drevets and his colleagues could see the brain areas where activity changed significantly during the anticipation of a touch-type sensation. The computer programs used in the PET scanners translated measurements of increased blood flow into different colors. The brighter, or "hotter," the color appearing in a part of the brain slice imaged in the computer screen, the greater the blood flow in that area. And, by inference, the harder that area of the brain was working.

When the volunteers waited for another gentle touch to their big toe, the blood flow in the parts of the somatosensory cortex devoted to the face and the fingers clearly decreased. At the same time, the PET scans showed that blood flow to the areas of the somatosensory cortex that processed touch data from the toes stayed the same as when the subjects were resting. This may at first seem confusing. What does the face have to do with the big toe? The answer lies not in the body parts themselves but in the somatosensory cortex. It turns out that the areas of the somatosensory cortex that handle sensations emanating from the skin on the face lie very close to the areas that deal with the toes.

The second experiment measured blood-flow changes in the brain while the volunteers anticipated an electric shock to their index finger. In this scenario, the PET scans showed that blood flow to the areas of the somatosensory cortex handling sensations in the fingers stayed the same. The blood flow to the regions dealing with sensory information from the face dropped considerably. Again, in the somatosensory cortex itself the regions that handle sensory data from the fingers lie close to those that deal with sensations coming from the face.

Finally, the snakes and tarantulas. The PET scans showed that blood flow decreased significantly to the regions of the somatosensory cortex that receive sensory information from the fingers. However, the parts of the somatosensory zones devoted to the lips stayed the same.

So what's all this mean? According to Drevets, these PET-scan images give us a look at how the brain's somatosensory cortex gets ready to handle an anticipated influx of sensory information. Essentially, the parts of the somatosensory cortex devoted to body areas not involved get "tuned out." At the same time, the somatosensory regions that handle the body area from which the sensory information is expected to come stay active and alert. The decreases in blood flow happened in those parts of the somatosensory cortex that surround the area which would handle the anticipated sensation. Drevets and his colleagues speculate that this suppression of activity in those regions handling sensations from places on the skin where no stimulus is expected may improve the transmission of the anticipated stimulus through the appropriate sensory pathways.

However, nothing is as simple as it seems when it comes to the brain. Several researchers doing somewhat similar experiments with visual perception have found *increases* in blood flow to relevant parts of the somatosensory cortex. In those studies, unlike the one carried out by Drevets, the subjects really did experience the anticipated stimuli. That could explain the difference.

Two other difficulties also arise in interpreting the PET-scan data from the Drevets experiments. First, the changes in blood flow in the brain that PET scans measure are caused by the activity taking place at the synapses of millions of neurons. Some of those synapses are inhibitory; they suppress activity in the neurons to which they connect. Others are excitatory, causing the next neurons in line to fire off. PET scans don't discriminate between inhibitory and excitatory action. It's just activity. Researchers therefore still don't know how a decrease in blood flow in parts of the somatosensory cortex surrounding the "focus of attention" actually influences the activity of the neurons in that area. Are inhibitory synapses in the affected areas slowing down in activity, thus allowing the neurons in the focus area of the somatosensory cortex to become more active? Or is it more complex: Perhaps excitatory synapses in the affected areas connected to *inhibitory synapses* in the focus area are being shut down. Would that in turn slow down the inhibitory synapses in the focus area of somatosensory cortex to which they are connected, allowing that area to become really attentive? No one knows yet.

The second difficulty has to do with PET's inherent slowness. Forty seconds is a long, long time in the cosmos of the brain. As we saw in the last chapter, Alan Gevins and his enhanced EEG machines can detect and map activity in the brain happening on a time scale of milliseconds. It is possible to determine the time over which attention has an influence in the brain by using scalp electrodes of an EEG to measure electrical activity in the brain. Researchers can compare recordings taken while subjects pay attention (or "attend to") a sensory stimulus with those taken when they are not paying attention. The recordings measure *event potentials*—the minute changes in electrical activity that take place when a persons attention is aroused by some sensory stimulus. These experiments have shown increases and decreases in electrical activity caused by synaptic firing that take place on time scales of 100 milliseconds or so. The 40 seconds of a PET scan is four-hundred times as long as the flickering change in brain activity taking place in just 100 milliseconds. So PET scans, as dramatic as they look and as valuable as they indeed are, nevertheless provide us with only a crude look at what is really taking place in the brain's somatosensory cortex.

THE MUSICAL BRAIN

Another sense that has gotten a lot of attention from researchers using the new brain-imaging technologies is the sense of hearing. The brain's two auditory cortexes lie atop the left and right temporal lobes, the outer parts of the brain sitting just behind the temples. It is here that the primary processing of auditory information takes place. The auditory cortex registers a sound's loudness, pitch, and timbre. Loudness corresponds to the strength of the sound waves that the ears have detected. The frequency of the sound waves, the number of waves per second, equals the sound's pitch. Timbre is a quality produced by the blending of several sounds from different voices, instruments, or other sources.

All this sound information arrives from the ears. The main purpose of the ears is to convert sound waves into electrochemical signals that will travel to the brain's auditory cortexes. This information gets from ear to brain in a fashion reminiscent of the old gospel song about "the thigh bone connected to the shin bone." The fleshy tunnel of the outer ear—the part we all see sticking out from the sides of our heads—channels sound waves into the middle ear. Here the sound waves strike the tiny sheet of tissue called the eardrum. The eardrum in turn transmits the sound vibrations to three tiny bones called the malleus ("the hammer"), the incus ("the anvil"), and the stapes ("the stirrup").

The sound wave causes the the tiny stapes (it's the smallest bone in the body) to plunge back and forth through the entry to the inner ear, called the oval window. Inside the inner ear is a system of fluid-filled chambers that are connected to the cochlea, a structure shaped like a snail shell. The movement of the stapes sends waves pulsing through the fluid in the cochlea, vibrating a membrane. This, in turn, causes vibrations in a long tube connected to the cochlea called the organ of Corti.*

---

*This thin spiral tube is named for its discoverer, the Italian anatomist Alfonso Corti (1822–88).

The organ of Corti is lined with thousands of tiny hairs, or cilia, which are attached to about thirty-thousand auditory nerve fibers.

Different cilia respond to vibrations of specific wavelengths, or particular strength or timbre, which is ultimately how the auditory cortex distinguishes these features. When the cilia vibrate, they activate the neurons to which they are attached. And that's how sound waves get turned into electrochemical signals transmitted through neurons to the brain.

As the auditory signals from the ears travel through the nerve fibers, they first go to the brain stem, part of the brain lying just above the top of the spinal cord. There they pass through several different neural relay stations. Some of the nerves from the left ear cross over to the right auditory cortex and vice versa. Others do not cross over and connect directly to the left auditory cortex. The same is true of some nerve fibers coming from the right ear. Thus, signals from both ears get processed in both the right and left auditory cortex. If you should suffer damage to one auditory cortex from an injury or a stroke, you will not necessarily become deaf in the opposite ear.

All the brain does with auditory information in the auditory cortexes is give it some primary processing and categorizing. At this point it is just sound. Noise. For sound to have meaning, other parts of the brain must come into play. As we'll see in more detail in chapter 10, two areas in the brain's left hemisphere play an important role in turning sound into speech.

But what about music? Several researchers over the years have suggested that music is largely processed in the right cerebral hemisphere. For example, Michael Phelps of UCLA, one of the inventors of PET, produced several PET images showing active right auditory cortexes in people who were listening to music. However, the evidence for this right-hemisphere laterality has been fragmentary and often contradicted by other studies showing areas in the left temporal lobe involved in musical appreciation.

Music and spoken language do have something very important in common: Both are rhythmic. Considerable evidence now exists that the brain is predisposed to detect patterns—in sound, in vision, in touch, in every form of sensory information that comes into it. And that makes sense. It is by detecting patterns that the brain is able to create (or detect) order in the welter of data that constantly floods it. The auditory cortexes compare the multitude of sound signals coming into them, sorting them out and grouping them into orderly patterns that correspond to pitch, loudness, and timbre.

For auditory data to be understood as speech or deciphered and appreciated as music, they have to get from the auditory cortex to these so-called higher-order processing regions in the left and right hemispheres. It is in these regions that sound becomes words, phrases, or sentences. The words, phrases, and sentences are imbued with symbolic meaning, and language as we know it takes place. It is in these regions that sound becomes patterns of notes, musical phrases, sonatas, symphonies. But the question is still asked: Is it in the right or left hemisphere that music is processed? Or both? Or somewhere else?

MOST PEOPLE associate Ravel's name with "Bolero," and its use in the movie *10*. But Ravel was a composer famous in his field for much more than that fascinating melody. Along with Claude Debussy, Ravel was a leading exponent of musical Impressionism and within the structure of classical forms composed highly original and fluid music. Among his most famous works for piano are *Le Tombeau de Couperin* and *Valses Nobles et Sentimentales* and the orchestral work *Rhapsodie Espagnole*.

Several years before his death in 1937, Ravel was in an automobile accident that severely injured his brain's left hemisphere. He gradually developed a progressive condition that robbed him of many basic motor skills as well as the ability to write. Worse, he later lost his ability to compose, read, sing in tune, or even play music. It must have been a terrible blow to this incredibly creative man. Despite these losses, Ravel could still play scales on the piano; he could also hear musical pieces "in his head." Nor did he ever lose his feelings of joy and pleasure at listening to music, which he did avidly until his death.

In 1992 psychologist Justine Sergent, of McGill University in Montreal, and her colleagues published the results of a set of experiments that have a direct bearing on Ravel's tragic condition. The experiments do so by providing the first real clues to the regions of the brain that are actually involved in musical performance. Sergent and her colleagues used PET and MRI scans to study the working brains of ten right-handed classical pianists, each with at least fifteen years of experience tickling the ivories. What she found was that a whole network of areas in the brain are set into action when a pianist reads musical notation and plays it on a keyboard.

Sergent first took some baseline PET measurements. One set was done while the volunteers were resting and looking at a blank screen; another, while each person responded with finger or hand movements to a pattern of dots on the screen; and finally, while each volunteer listened to and played some musical scales. Next, she and her colleagues did PET scans one minute long while each volunteer reclined and read a musical score written for the right hand. Then they carried out another set of one-minute PET scans while each volunteer played the same score on a small electronic keyboard near at hand.

By using a computer to subtract the baseline brain images from the experimental sets, the researchers could isolate the areas that were actually involved in the two tasks they had carried out. Then Sergent superimposed the resulting PET images on MRI images previously made of the volunteers' brains. MRI produces extremely clear images of the brain's physical structure, something PET cannot do well. The resulting composite images made it possible to really pinpoint the brain regions with greatest blood flow and thus the greatest activity during the tests.

Sergent and her associates found that sight-reading musical scores and actually playing the music both activate regions in all four of the cortex's lobes—frontal, temporal, parietal, and occipital. Parts of the cerebellum, which lies near the back and bottom of the brain, are also activated during these tasks. Some of the neural clusters that are part of this "music network" lie right next to some areas involved in processing words in the left cerebral hemisphere—but are not the same. Sergent also found that some brain areas activated in the tests appear to handle the spatial information symbolized by notes on a musical staff. And that might explain Maurice Ravel's loss of musical ability after his auto accident. The area of his left hemisphere damaged in the crash must have been one that was a part of the brain's musical network.

The combined MRI-PET images provide the first real look at areas in the brain that are clearly associated with music. But Sergent herself, in a 1992 interview, sounded a note of caution. She pointed out that sight-reading and piano playing are only a small part of the whole musical experience. "We are still far from understanding the pleasure and emotions elicited by music," she added.

ANOTHER RESEARCHER who has been studying the brain's musical connections is Gottfried Schlaug, a neurologist at Heinrich Heine University in Düsseldorf, Germany, and a research fellow in neurology at Beth Israel Hospital in Boston, Massachusetts. In recent years Schlaug has looked at the phenomenon of perfect pitch, as well as the differences between trained musicians and nonmusicians.

In 1993, Schlaug and his colleagues in Düsseldorf looked for possible differences and similarities between the brain structures of musicians and nonmusicians. They worked with fifty-four volunteers; half were classically trained, right-handed male piano or string players, and the other half were right-handed male nonmusicians. The researchers carried out a series of MRI scans of the volunteers' brains, taking advantage of MRI's excellence at creating images of brain structures.

Schlaug and his associates found some rather striking differences in the brains of their two groups of subjects. One difference had to do with a small neural structure in the cerebral cortex that processes sound signals. It is called the planum temporale. In the professional musicians this structure was larger in the left hemisphere and smaller in the right than in the brains of the nonmusicians.

Another difference was in the corpus callosum. This is the thick, long band of nerve tissue lying at the base of the forebrain that connects similar parts of the left and right cerebral hemispheres. (It's the reason, by the way, that we have only one brain, not a "left brain" and a "right brain." The corpus callosum allows the brain's two hemispheres to constantly communicate with one another.) The musicians had a thicker corpus callosum than did the nonmusicians. The difference was especially evident in those musicians who had begun their training as young children. In these adults, the corpus callosum was 10–15 percent thicker than in nonmusicians, or even musicians who started training late in childhood.

As we saw in chapter 4, the brain of an infant or child is a veritable learning machine. The more it learns, the more neural connections it creates, and the denser the brain becomes. Nerve tracts and fibers that are involved in these processes also become thicker, in general. One result of this discovery is that learning specialists the world over are now urging that schools and other educational institutions find ways to really help children "grow their brains." Schlaug's findings seem to corroborate this position. He feels that his MRI images reveal that early musical training physically shapes and molds the young brain. It strengthens existing neural connections and probably adds new ones. The thicker corpus callosum, he speculates, may help the motor cortex do a better job of coordinating the complex motor movements needed to play a difficult piece of music. As for the larger planum temporale, the brain's sound-signal processor, Schlaug suspected that it plays a role in overall musical ability, including a better "ear" for pitch, timbre, and intonation.

This, in turn, leads into Schlaug's interest in the musical gift of perfect pitch. Perhaps 1 percent or less of the general population has the ability to hear a single musical note and immediately know its pitch. Most people can tell the difference between two musical notes when they have heard them both and can thus mentally compare them. If the notes are sufficiently far apart on the scale, almost anyone can tell they are different in pitch. Some people, however, are tone-deaf. They may not be able to sing any musical note that is not similar to sounds they use in speaking. Others can tell that there is a difference between two notes but cannot determine which is higher and which is lower in pitch. At the other end of the scale are those people with perfect pitch. They will know at once that one note is middle C, another is D above high C, and that still another is A-flat below middle C. Perfect pitch appears to be almost impossible to learn formally later in life. It seems to be connected to either a genetic predisposition, very early exposure to music, or possibly a combination of both.

In research published in *Science* magazine in 1995, Schlaug and several colleagues reported on their efforts to zero in on the brain's sound-signal processor, the planum temporale. Their previous work had already shown that this structure in the left cerebral hemisphere of musicians was larger than that in nonmusicians. This particular kind of functional asymmetry had been a bit unexpected. Other studies, including the one done by McGill's Justine Sergent, suggested that the right hemisphere might be dominant for musical processing. Schlaug's interest in this region was also heightened by his discovery of a study done back in the 1950s of a German musician who had suffered a stroke and experienced melody deafness.

In his new study, Schlaug wanted to determine what, if any, differences in the brain's sound-signal processor existed between professional musicians with perfect pitch, those without perfect pitch, and nonmusicians without perfect pitch.

Once again, Schlaug and his associates used MRI to probe the brains of their subjects. The MRI images confirmed some of Schlaug's earlier findings. The brain's sound-signal processor in the left cerebral hemisphere was larger than the one in the right hemisphere. This was true for both musicians and nonmusicians. What's more, the difference in size was twice as great for musicians as for the nonmusicians. Simple statistical analysis revealed that nearly all of this huge disparity was caused by the presence of the perfect-pitch people in the musician group. In other words, their left planum temporales were extraordinarily large.

As many as 95 percent of all musicians with perfect pitch start their musical training before the age of seven—a powerful argument for the role of learning in the development of this gift. Schlaug and his associates also discovered that those musicians without perfect pitch who began their training when they were older children had no greater asymmetry of their planum temporales than did the nonmusicians. At the same time, considerable evidence exists that perfect pitch runs in families, with half the children apparently inheriting this gift. So genetics must play some significant role as well.

Despite Schlaug's fascinating findings, disagreement still reigns in this field. Robert Zatorre, a cognitive neuroscientist at the Montreal Neurological Institute (the same organization where Justine Sergent worked), has done research showing that music is primarily processed in the brain's right auditory cortex, not in the left cerebral hemisphere. In particular, a study by Zatorre and his colleagues published in a 1994 issue of the prestigious *Journal of Neuroscience* suggests that areas in the right cerebral hemisphere are activated when a person listens to a melody he or she has not heard before. Zatorre has said that his research consistently shows that parts of the right auditory cortex play a vital role in listening to musical patterns and determining whether pitch is going up or down. If a person has a stroke that affects these parts of the right auditory cortex, Zatorre has said, that person can easily lose some of the ability to appreciate music without losing all musical ability. Individuals who suffer strokes that damage both sides of the brain where sounds are processed can easily lose all ability to appreciate music. In one case, for example, one of Zatorre's patients with that kind of damage could no longer tell the difference between classical music, jazz, and rap.

But is there really a controversy here? Perhaps not. Zatorre has suggested that his and Schlaug's findings are more complementary than contradictory. That is, each researcher may be looking at different aspects of the same neurological phenomenon. The right cerebral hemisphere and its auditory cortex may be involved in processing some aspects of music, while the left hemisphere handles others. As we'll see in chapter 10, even spoken languages appear to be handled in an analogous fashion. At least one researcher has found tiny regions in both the left and right cerebral cortex that process different parts of spoken language.

One of Schlaug's colleagues at Beth Israel Hospital thinks this may be the case. Dr. Albert Galaburda thinks that pitch—including perfect pitch—is processed in the left hemisphere. This is because perceiving pitch requires both verbal and musical skills. It is no coincidence, he feels, that the left planum temporale just happens to include a part of Wernicke's area, the part of the brain that makes language comprehension possible. Verbal associations take place when a person with perfect pitch identifies a single note. In essence, that person is either saying aloud or silently, "That's middle C; that's D below high C; that's A-flat above middle C."

Schlaug himself agrees that this may be the case. He has said that the processing of much of music's overall melodic components may take place in the right hemisphere, while the task of identifying pitch and naming notes occurs in the brain's sound signal processor in the left hemisphere.

Still, a major question remains unanswered: *Why* is music processing, particularly pitch processing, so asymmetrical? One possible answer has to do with speed. No matter how thick your corpus callosum, neural signals just take less time to travel from one *part* of a cerebral hemisphere to another part than from one cerebral hemisphere to the other. And quicker signal transmission time means more efficient processing of the data by the brain.

One postscript to this excursion into the brain's musical connection: Gottfried Schlaug does not have perfect pitch. But he used to be a very good organist.

PET, MRI, EEG, and other imaging technologies have been put to use studying all the many senses we possess. Touch and hearing are only two that have begun yielding their secrets to the researchers and their brain scanners. However, the sense that has historically received the most attention from brain researchers has been sight. This has been no less the case during the Decade of the Brain than it has for the last century. As we'll soon see, our new images of visual perception are throwing new light on how the brain perceives the world and how it also creates the world within itself.

CHAPTER 7

VISUALIZING THE WORLD

ONLY IN THE LAST ten years or so have my parents begun wearing glasses, and then only for reading. Like many people who have had normal sight most of their lives, they started getting somewhat farsighted in their later years. It's not uncommon, and it has nothing to do with the brain's visual-perception apparatus. The lens in the eye starts losing its elasticity, and it is harder to focus on objects close to one's face, like a book or newspaper. My mother has also started having problems with glaucoma; in fact, she has pretty much lost all sharp vision in one eye. Again, this is a problem that develops in the eye itself, not in the brain.

Several of their children—including me—are nearsighted. In my case, I've worn glasses since I was seven years old and contact lenses for about three years. I am extremely nearsighted, with two very elongated eyeballs. This physiological stretching of the eyeballs has steadily increased over time, and my nearsightedness has grown slowly worse. In the spring of 1995 it led to a far more serious condition. The retina in my right eye tore loose in what my ophthalmologist called "a giant retinal tear." Several surgeries and laser treatments later, the vision in my right eye is still crippled. It may well never be the same; in fact, I could still lose all sight in that eye.

One of the signs of serious trouble that occurred early in this ongoing battle for my right eye was the appearance of light flashes. Unexpectedly, for no apparent reason, I would see sudden lightninglike flashes of light in the lower left part of my right eye's visual field. This was quite a startling experience. At first, I didn't know what was going on; I naturally thought I was seeing some kind of flash of light coming from "out there." From the outer world. A glint of the sun off a car's side-view mirror? Sunlight through a window? But then, at night, as I lay in bed, I saw the flashes again. My eyes were closed. Something very strange was going on. I later discovered that light flashes of this kind are common when one has suffered a detached retina. The trauma causes the neurons in the retina that ordinarily react to light coming in from the outside to instead spontaneously send erroneous signals to the brain's visual cortex.

The brain can't possibly "know" that these signals are *not* caused by normal external stimuli. So it interprets them as it has learned to interpret all such information. In my case, I thought I was seeing flashes from light hitting the inner left quadrant of my right eye's visual field. In fact, the signals were generated by a part of the damaged retina in the *upper-right corner* of my right eye. The brain inverts the visual signals coming from the eyes, so we see the world right side up instead of upside down. Even if the signal is generated *inside* the eye itself, the brain will "invert" the information. What was happening on my right eye's right side, the brain "saw" happening on the left side.

Which leads one to repeat the question once asked in song by the famous rock-and-roll band the Moody Blues: "What is real / and what *is* an illusion?"

It's a good question, one that still has no answer. However, many researchers are now using the latest noninvasive brain-imaging technologies to discover what the brain does as it processes sensory information. We are learning more than ever before about how our brains smell, taste, hear, feel—and, especially, see.

THE EYE AND HOW IT SEES

One of the major goals of neuroscientists and cognitive scientists has been to understand how the brain receives, stores, processes, and interprets all this information. In pursuit of this goal, they study all the body's senses. However, our visual sense has far and away received the most attention from brain researchers. More than any other sense, our eyes provide us with the greatest amount of detailed information about our environment. Vision's paramount role is reflected in the brain. In both birds and primates, classes of animal that rely heavily on sight, the areas of the brain that deal with vision are much larger and more complex than the areas devoted to the other senses. For example, the auditory nerve, which runs from the ear to the brain, contains about thirty-thousand nerve fibers. The optic nerve, running from the eye to the brain, contains some 2 million nerve fibers. That's sixty times as many as the main auditory nerve.

What's more, as much as 30 percent of the human cerebral cortex is probably involved in processing information coming back from the visual cortex at the rear of the brain. These so-called higher areas of the brain include parts of an "association cortex" located in the parietal lobes, which stretch from the top of the brain toward the back of the head. They also include the decision-making regions of the frontal lobes at the front of the brain, just behind the forehead. These regions take the data provided by the visual cortex and turn them into what we are *aware* of seeing. Here, in some mysterious way, the brain connects the visual data with concept data. I see trees, forests; the bloom of the rose and the deer eating the roses; my mother's face, my mother.

NEARLY EVERY creature on earth possesses some sort of visual sense. Even some single-celled creatures have regions sensitive to light. Plants and flowers are also sensitive to the presence or absence of light. These kinds of light-sensitive cells do not form images. But as we begin moving up the evolutionary ladder, we begin encountering creatures with visual senses that do see images of the world around them. Primates have remarkably complex eyes. Humans have complex eyes connected to complex brains.

Because our eyes face forward from the front of the skull, we have binocular vision. Binocular vision equals true perspective, a three dimensional view of the world.

Six muscles move our eyes about and help hold them in their sockets. Our eyes move in a rapid sequence of tiny stops and starts. At each brief pause, they sample the visual data from the outside world. The brain compensates for the jerking movements and eliminates any blurring in the final images. In fact, considerable evidence now exists that the brain samples all the incoming visual data in frames of about a tenth of a second each. The brain then combines all the "frames" into a smooth vision of reality. It is as if the brain images the outer world the way a movie camera does, in discrete frames. Our experience of a seamlessly perceived world is as much an illusion as the smoothly moving images on the motion-picture screen.

Each adult human eye is about an inch in diameter. It consists of several layers of tissue, some cavities filled with watery or jellylike substances, and the structures that actually make vision possible. They include the cornea and lens, which focus light to a point; the iris and its pupil, which help sharpen vision and adapt to the intensity of light; and the retina, which is the eye's "photographic film."

First comes the cornea, the clear, curved surface at the very front of the eye. This is the eye's first and most important focusing mechanism. The cornea's curved surface and general composition make it act like a lens.*

The light that has passed through the cornea traverses a small chamber filled with clear fluid. It then passes through the pupil, a hole at the center of a circular membrane called the iris. Two sets of muscles in the iris expand and contract the membrane, opening the pupil or closing it to a tiny pinhole. Information about the amount of light hitting the retina at the back of the eye gets sent to the brain. The brain then interprets that information and sends impulses back to the iris muscles. Too much light and the iris contracts. Too little light and the iris dilates. The iris's action also helps focus and sharpen the image.

The light travels through another tiny chamber behind the iris and its pupil and passes through the lens. Like the cornea, the lens is made of fine, clear fibers. The lens has a convex shape; it looks like a left and right parenthesis nestled together. By contrast, a concave lens looks like a right and left parenthesis sitting side by side. The lens of the eye acts like a typical convex glass lens in a microscope or telescope. Light passing through the cornea and lens is bent to a point, and the distance from the lens to the focal point is called the focal length (Fig. 7.1).

Two sets of muscles attached to the lens change its shape and affect its ability to focus light. This allows the eye to focus on objects lying at different distances. As a person ages, the elasticity of the lens decreases, causing the lens's convex sides to flatten a bit. The result is the most common form of farsightedness, an inability to see near objects clearly.

---

*The cornea's degree of curvature is important. If the curvature is not the same at all points on its surface, the image coming into the eye will be distorted. This condition is called astigmatism. As we get older, the tissue of the cornea begins to get "flabby" and starts to relax. That's why astigmatism is a common condition in older people.

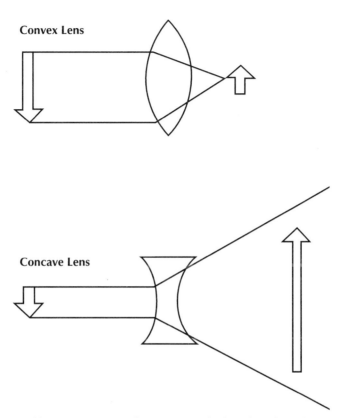

Fɪɢ. 7.1.   Two types of lenses, convex and concave, and what they do to light.

This is the reason my parents—now in their vigorous seventies—have become farsighted. Light entering their eyes tends to hit a focal point lying behind the retina. Farsightedness is also caused by an eyeball that is a bit too short. By contrast, nearsightedness is an inability to see distant objects clearly. It is caused by an eyeball that is too elongated or a lens and cornea that focus light at a point in front of the retina.

The beam of focused light from the outer world now crosses a large chamber filled with a clear, jellylike substance and falls upon the retina. The image painted upon the retina is small—10 microns, or 0.0003937 inch across under ideal conditions. But it is here, on and within the retina, that the real magic of vision begins.

FROM THE RETINA TO THE BRAIN

Lining the inner walls of the eyeball is the retina. Along with the optic nerve to which it is connected, the retina is essentially part of the brain. It is the only part of the central nervous system that can be directly observed in a living creature. The retina is a thin structure of remarkable complexity and consists of four layers of cells and two layers of cell connections. Contained in these layers are five different types of neurons.

The part of the retina we actually see with, called the photoreceptive layer, contains two types of specialized, light-sensitive neurons called *rods* and *cones*. Each human eye contains about 125 million rods and cones. Five percent of them, about 6 million, are cones, but their importance far outweighs their numbers. The cone cells are responsible for color vision. Different types of cones are "tuned" to different wavelengths of light. Physicists know that "color" (more accurately, hue) is purely a function of the wavelength of light. The longer the wavelength, the "redder" the light we perceive. The shorter the wavelength, the "bluer" the light.

Most humans have three types of cones containing three different chemical pigments. Each pigment absorbs light of a different wavelength. These three cones are called the blue, green, and red cones.

This is the classic explanation of color vision. However, it turns out that human color vision is not quite as simple and clear-cut as everyone has assumed. Some people with normal color vision have two different types of red cones. Others have slightly different varieties of the green cones. And some folks have different versions of both red and green cones. Each of these variants is sensitive to a slightly different part of the color spectrum—to different shades of green and red. So the retina can actually contain up to five possible types of cones, containing as many as five different kinds of chemical pigments.

Despite these variations, these people perceive color in exactly the same way everyone else does. It doesn't seem to matter to the brain what version of the red or green cone a person has in his or her retina. Apparently, similar types of cones "pool" their color data. Three primary colors create all possible colors, and the brain somehow knows this. It is able to combine the variations in color sensitivity of the two different red and green cones and end up with the standard "red" and "green" that everyone perceives.

Cones also play another important role in the retina. At a point on the retina near the rear of the eye is a spot called the macula. Within the macula lutea is a tiny depression less than a hundredth of a square millimeter in area. This part of the retina, called the fovea, contains about 2,000 cones arranged in a hexagonal array. They are so tightly packed that the fovea has an effective density of 150,000 cones per square millimeter. The fovea is thus the area of most acute vision, and the eye takes advantage of this fact. The eyes "paint" an image of interest onto the fovea so that its finest details can be detected. The shape of the lens even changes so that the sharpest image possible focuses on the fovea. We have all had the experience of having our eyes "riveted" on an object of intense interest. Perhaps it is the face of our lover or a slight movement in the trees that signals the presence of a deer we are hunting. Whatever that object might be, our brains tell our eyes to point at it in such a way that its image will fall directly on the fovea and its cluster of cone cells.

Cones function only at light levels typical of daylight. Rod cells, by contrast, are very sensitive to low light levels but cannot detect colors. When we turn out the lights in our house or apartment at night and go to bed, the room at first may seem pitch-black. Within a minute or so, though, we can again begin to discern the shapes of objects in the room, the door frame leading to the hallway, the shadowy shape of the curtains over the window. Something moves; a moment passes, and we recognize the dark shape as the cat on a nightly prowl of her domain. The world is painted in shades of gray, but it is the world. We see it because the rod cells in our retina detect even the low levels of light in the room.

The rods and cones connect to other nerve cells in the retina in a pattern as complex as some parts of the brain itself. The connections leading from the rods and cones eventually form the retina's nerve-fiber layer. The nerves in this layer converge at a point about 3 millimeters below the macula. Here they form a small whitish area on the retina totally lacking any rods or cones. This is the eye's *blind spot*, where the nerve fibers bundle together to form the optic nerve. This is the only spot on a healthy retina that cannot "see." Because there are no rods or cones in the blind spot, it is truly blind.

The hundreds of millions of cells in the retina detect the photons, encode the data into electrical impulses, and send them on their way to the brain. Rods and cones play an important role, but so do the other neurons in the retina. In particular, many of the other neurons in the retina carry out different "filtering" functions. The 125 million rods and cones ultimately connect to the million neuronal fibers in each optic nerve. Try forcing the water flowing through a water main 1 meter wide directly into a garden hose 2 centimeters in diameter. It can't be done without blowing out the hose. To prevent that from happening to the optic nerve, most of the raw visual data from the retina gets filtered out.

The filtering process is by no means spread equally across the retina. For example, everything the fovea detects goes to the optic nerve and on to the brain. At the outer parts of the retina, though, only one bit of data per thousand or more will get through. All of this happens *in the retina, in the eye itself*. This is how the retina acts like sophisticated brain tissue, sacrificing resolving power in favor of high sensitivity to the most important parts of an image.

Once visual information leaves the eyes via the optic nerves, it takes a strange and still somewhat mysterious journey to the very back of brain. The *primary visual cortex* lies at the rear of the occipital lobe. Figure 7.2 shows that neural impulses from the left and right eyes cross to the opposite hemispheres, but in a somewhat complex fashion. At a region below and at the back of the frontal lobes called the optic chiasma, the optic nerves cross over in a way that causes this split to take place. Remember, the lenses in the eyes have inverted the light. So the visual image being formed on the retina is both upside down and reversed left to right.

The signals now travel through a set of nerve fibers called the optic tract. The fibers of the optic tract then fan out into another set of nerve fibers and finally arrive in the primary visual cortex. The result: Information from the right half of *each eye's* visual field goes to the primary visual cortex in the right cerebral hemisphere, and information from each eye's left visual field gets piped to the left cerebral hemisphere's primary visual cortex.

Each cell in the primary visual cortex receives input from a particular location on the retina. This means that there is a precise relationship between locations on the retina and locations in the visual cortex. The visual cortex itself is thus a kind of neural map of the retinas.

The retina has its highest concentration of neurons at the center of our fields of vision. Information from that part of the eye travels to the backmost part of the visual cortex. A relatively huge number of neurons process this most important visual data. Neural impulses from areas of the retina that lie farther and farther away from the center of the visual

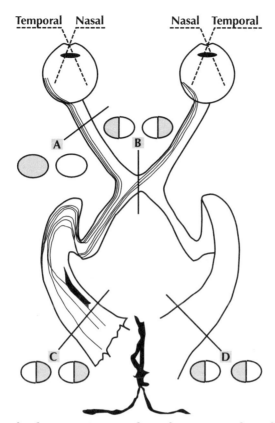

Temporal Nasal   Nasal Temporal

Fig. 7.2.   Visual information coming from the eyes travels to the back of the brain by a complex route. Neural impulses from the right visual field of each eye pass through the optic nerves (A). In the optic chiasma (B) some nerve fibers cross over, so that information from the two left visual fields ends up in the left side of the primary visual cortex (C). Impulses from the right visual fields go to the right side of the primary visual cortex (D).

fields are progressively mapped to neuron clusters that lie farther forward in the visual cortex.

Running from left to right along the back of the occipital lobe at the rear of the brain, and the visual cortex, which is a part of it, is a prominent groove, or wrinkle, in the cortex. Information from the upper half of each eye's visual field goes to regions in the visual cortex lying below this groove, while data from the lower part of each visual field end up in parts of the visual cortex above the groove.

MAPPING THE BRAIN'S VISION CENTER

Marcus Raichle is one of the pioneers and leading experts in the use of positron-emission tomography (PET) to probe the living brain. Early on in the use of PET for brain imaging, Raichle quickly realized he could test its accuracy by using it to probe this known topographic organization of the primary visual cortex.

He and his colleagues showed several volunteers a series of pictures on a TV monitor and monitored their brain's blood flow with a PET scanner. The image they used was a red-and-black annular checkerboard (a circular checkerboard with a hole in the middle) with a tiny white dot in the center. The volunteers were to keep their eyes focused on the white dot. By varying its size on the monitor, the researchers could "paint" the image right onto their foveas—the most sensitive part of the retina—or onto areas near the fovea or parts of the retina lying far away from the fovea. The control readings were made with the subjects looking at the monitor while there was only a white dot. By subtracting the computerized PET images made during the control runs from those made during the actual tests, Raichle and his colleagues could isolate just those parts of the visual cortex that were activated.

The results were exactly in line with what brain researchers already knew about the visual cortex. The very tiny annular checkerboards painted their images right onto the fovea. When the subjects were looking at these images, the rearmost parts of the visual cortex "lit up" in the computerized PET images. As the checkerboard pictures got larger and moved farther out from the fovea, the active brain areas moved progressively forward in the visual cortex.

Next, Raichle showed the checkerboard pictures to a second group of people in a way that painted the image onto either the upper or lower half of their visual fields. Once again, the PET scans showed the active areas of the brain moving from below to above the calcarine sulcus.

Finally, the researchers showed the checkerboard to first the right and then the left sides of the volunteers' visual fields. Again, the results followed their predictions. The PET images showed the lit-up active parts of the brain moving from the left to the right primary visual cortex as the checkerboard picture shifted from the right to the left visual field.

This was not a new discovery, but it was still an important piece of research. It proved that PET was a highly accurate method of probing the functional activity of the human brain. It also laid the groundwork for a whole series of research projects that Raichle and other brain researchers have carried out since then on the brain and its activity during vision and language.

IMAGINARY SCENES

One of those researchers is Stephen Kosslyn, a psychologist at Harvard University. Kosslyn is interested in mental imagery as well as the nuts and bolts of the visual-perception system. Mental imagery is essentially the process by which a person conjures up visual images in his or her imagination.

Suppose, for example, that I ask you to close your eyes and imagine that you see a tree. You will promptly call up in your "mind's eye," or imagination, an image of a tree. Does it have leaves? I ask. Yes, you reply, and now your mental image of a tree has leaves. This is an apple tree, I continue. Let's make those leaves look like apple leaves. And so they do. The tree has some bright red apples hanging from it. In your imaginary picture of the tree, it now has apples.

These are the kinds of mental processes that have baffled brain researchers for years. How does the brain perform mental imagery? Does it use the same neural networks that normal vision uses or some other set of neural connections? And where is the mental image located, anyway? If you have carried out the mental task of imagining a tree, you have probably felt that you could almost see that picture in your head. It feels as if you have some kind of movie screen up there on which your imagination flashes its mental pictures.

According to Kosslyn and other researchers, evidence continues to mount that the brain makes mental images the same way it creates the images that arrive via the eyes—only backwards. In regular vision, the visual stimulus is first processed in the primary visual cortex at the back of the brain. From there the information gets passed through various nerve fibers to other regions of the brain for additional processing. If the image is of a letter or a word, language regions become involved. The brain's auditory cortex will play a role if sound stimuli are associated with the image. And so on, until regions in the brain's frontal lobe called the association cortex imbue the image with a sense of recognition.

When we fantasize an image, our brains essentially run the process backwards. The stimulus originates in the brain's higher centers, like the association cortex in the frontal lobe. Then the stimulus gets passed down to the primary visual cortex, where it is constructed into an image. So there is nothing "imaginary" about an imagined image of an apple tree. It is as real to the brain and as real *in* the brain as seeing that actual apple tree out in my backyard.

Kosslyn and his associates at Harvard have used PET scans to watch what happens in people's brains when they construct mental images. In one particular experiment, Kosslyn had his volunteer subjects carry out a simple task under two different conditions. In the first case, the subject sat in front of a computer screen showing a grid of squares. Each volunteer was asked to construct a mental image, then answer a question about that image and signal their arrival at an answer by pressing a button on a keypad. In the second situation, each volunteer was shown an image on the grid, asked a question about it, and was then required to produce the same response when he or she reached an answer. In this second task, the subjects were not forming a mental image by trying to imagine a capital F fitting into the grid pattern. They were actually looking at the F on the screen.

In a typical experiment, the first task for a volunteer would be to sit at the screen, look at a lowercase letter f, and then be asked to imagine an uppercase F fitting into the grid on the screen. In the second task, the uppercase F would already be on the grid. In both cases, the volunteer would then be asked to press the key when an "X" appeared on the screen at a location inside the "F" (Fig. 7.3). The volunteers also had their brains scanned while doing a control task. In this case, they would look at grids and X's on the computer screen but would simply press the button without making any mental decisions about anything.

By subtracting the readings taken during the control sessions, Kosslyn and his colleagues could see what parts of the brain lit up when the volunteers carried out the two experimental tasks. Kosslyn found that similar regions in the brain's temporal and parietal lobes were active in both cases. The parietal lobes, as we've seen, run from the top of the brain toward the back; the temporal lobes lie along the sides of the brain at about the location of our ears. It didn't matter if the people were imagining an F on the screen or actually seeing an F on the screen. Since the same parts of the brain were involved in creating a mental image of an F, the person could determine if the X was inside it.

AT ABOUT the same time that Kosslyn was carrying out this PET-scan experiment on vision at Harvard, Raichle and his colleagues Steven

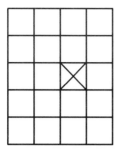

Task #1: Is the X inside the letter F?

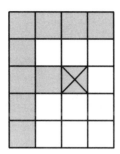

Task #2: Is the X inside the letter F?

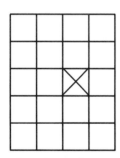

Control Task: No question asked.

FIG. 7.3.   The experimental setup for Stephen Kosslyn's study of visual imagery.

Petersen and Julies Fiez were doing something similar at Washington University. As in Kosslyn's experiment, the subjects also had two tasks to perform, and both were associated with letters. There was also a subtle but interesting difference. In Raichle's experiment, the subjects would first be shown a word written in uppercase letters, such as FIRE or CALM.

Then they would be asked to imagine if the lowercase version of the word contained an ascender. An ascender is a lowercase letter that has a part rising above the word's midline. The lowercase l is an ascender, for example. So is f. The uppercase word would stay on the computer screen for about 150 milliseconds before disappearing. The person would have about 2 seconds after this to recall the word from memory, decide if it contained an ascender, and then press a button if it did. Then the next uppercase word would appear.

The second task was similar to the first but differed in one important respect. In this task, the subjects would *listen* to a word and then have a moment to decide if it contained an ascender.

Raichle's results were remarkably similar to those of Kosslyn and his team. Raichle's PET images also showed the temporal and parietal lobes lighting up with furious activity as the person imagines the word he or she has just seen as written in lowercase letters and tries to picture if any of them are ascenders. The PET images taken when the subjects listened to the word have an interesting difference. In these images, the temporal lobes are not nearly as active as in the first task. Raichle thinks this suggests that temporal lobes are involved in changing an uppercase word that has been perceived *visually* into an imagined lowercase version. However, the parietal lobes are active in both situations. They play a role in this process whether the person hears or sees the word to be imaginatively transformed.

"WHAT," "WHERE," AND THE APPLE TREE

Raichle, Kosslyn, and other brain researchers now believe they are getting a good idea of what is happening in the brain when a person sees an object, and when that person imagines an image of the same object. Here's how it appears to work:

When you see the apple tree in my backyard, the sensory information from your retinas first travels to the primary visual system in the occipital lobe at the back of your brain. The primary visual system acts as what Kosslyn has called a "visual buffer." Here the image is almost literally mapped onto the neurons, just as it appears in the real world. This is probably the closest we get to having an inner eye or a mind's eye in our brains.

The visual cortex carries out an essential analysis of the image. Specific rows and columns of neurons in the visual cortex react only to lines at specific angles, for example. So the visual cortex analyzes the image in terms of line, contours, shadows, edges, depth of field, color, and other characteristics. The visual cortex examines each of these characteristics separately. At this point in the process of visual perception, the brain does not "know" that it is looking at an apple tree.

Next, says Kosslyn, specific features of the image get sent to two other areas of the brain. These areas are often referred to as the "what" and "where" subsystems. In order to identify the object, the brain must compare it with all the data it possesses about similar objects. It must also identify the object's location in three-dimensional space.

The temporal lobes along the side of the brain are part of the what subsystem. Here are found specific subsets of neurons that respond to impulses from other neurons, impulses that correspond to specific shapes and colors of objects. One such object is the "tree" shape, in all its nearly infinite variations. Another is the "leaf" shape, again with an enormous number of possible varieties of colors and shapes. None of these shapes, stored in the long-term-memory neural networks of the temporal lobes, have any specific location "in space." They are like templates of objects.

The where subsystem is found in the parietal lobes. Here are neurons that respond to objects in specific locations in space. If the tree shape is in the distance, for example, one set of neurons fires off. If it is up close, just at the end of my back porch, another set of neurons will fire. With this kind of knowledge, the brain can tell the body to move to the left to avoid walking into the tree.

Kosslyn thinks that once the what and where subsystems have done their work, the visual information travels to two more parts of the brain. One is a region in the occipital lobe at the rear of the brain where "associative memories" are stored. These are pieces of information associated with certain stimuli. If I see a eucalyptus leaf, I immediately recall its distinctive odor. That's an associative memory. Associated with the image of an apple may be smells, tastes, memories of the family kitchen when you were a child, the image of an apple pie, and so on. Signals from the what and where subsystems travel to the associative memory areas back in the occipital lobe. If good matches are made there, the brain recognizes the object you are looking at as an "apple tree."

But suppose the tree is quite a distance away, down the block or two backyards over. You cannot identify it simply from cues stored in associative memory. Now the brain sends the impulses to another subsys-

tem. They travel to the frontal lobes. It is here that the brain's sophisticated decision-making networks reside. The frontal lobes may contain
specific memories or information that allow you to identify the tree.
Perhaps it is the specific shape of the tree itself or the fact that it is *two*
backyards away, which puts it in, yes, my backyard. My wife and I have
an apple tree in our backyard. *Voilà!* The connection is made. Now the
signals travel down neural pathways back to the visual cortex, and your
brain identifies the object as an apple tree.

Brain researchers now know that every part of the brain that sends
visual information to other subsystems also receives information from
those same areas. A constant flow of information is taking place between
and among all these regions. It goes on continually.

And that, say Kosslyn and Raichle, is the reason why mental imagery
is what it is. The same process takes place as in seeing, but in reverse.
Instead of a physical, visual stimulus activating the set of neural pathways and networks, some other stimulus sets it off. This could be a
memory of your most recent visit to our house, for example. Or perhaps
the smell of that apple pie baking in the oven triggers the recollection of
the apple tree. It could be a song that comes on the oldies radio station—"Don't sit under the apple tree with anyone else but me. . . ."
Maybe it's a news report about the Andrews Sisters that recalls to your
mind the appletree song, which in turn triggers the memory of my apple
tree. Whatever. Now the impulses travel from your associative-memory
regions outward to the parietal and temporal lobes, activating the where
and what subsystems. From there the impulses move on to the primary
visual cortex to activate the neural maps at the back of your brain. The
neural columns and rows fire off. The image is created.

None of this happens instantly, of course, any more than visual perception happens at once. The more complex the mental image you are
creating, the longer the brain takes to build it up in the visual cortex.
Earlier I asked you to imagine a tree, then its leaves, and then the
apples. At each step the brain had to retrieve stored images from the
what or where subsystems, from the associational cortex, or from other
regions of the brain. Then the data had to travel back to the visual cortex to be incorporated into the image. Kosslyn's work with PET scans
has led him to estimate that each such step takes about .075 second.

It's important to realize that both these processes happen in the
brain simultaneously. The information constantly flows in both directions. Dramatic evidence for this comes from the experiences of some

stroke patients. One such person is a woman known in the medical literature as E.H. After suffering a stroke, this woman had a number of problems, including a very interesting change in her visual perception. She suffered from *achromatopsia*. Achromatopsia is, essentially, total loss of the ability to perceive color. E.H. could not *see* colors. The world now existed in various shades of gray for her. Even more fascinating: E.H. could not even *imagine* colors. When she recalled an object from memory, even one she had seen before her stroke, she could not tell you what color it was. In her mind's eye the object had no color. She could not conjure up a color in her memory or imagination.

The explanation for this has to do with the dual flow of visual information in the brain. E.H. lost the ability to *see* colors in objects she was perceiving in real time because of damage to the connections between the visual cortex and the brain's higher-level processing centers. That same damage prevented the opposite flow of information, from the what and where regions and the associative cortex back to the visual cortex. So she couldn't imagine colors, either.

THE BINDING PROBLEM

The what and where subsystems are just two of many in the brain that play a vital role in visual perception. For many years now, brain researchers have known or at least strongly suspected this to be the case. For example, in 1988 David Hubel published an article in *Science* that identified more than twenty such visual regions in the brains of primates, such as monkeys and humans. Other researchers put the number at around thirty or more. As we've already seen, the brain's primary visual cortex analyzes an image's specific features in distinct regions: Color, shape, shadows, and edges are all represented in specific cortical regions. Other areas outside the visual cortex help determine both what and where an object is.

If this is the case—and it surely is—then how does the brain put all this information together to create a unified perception of the object? Of all objects? Of the entire world outside the brain? I look at my father as he sits in his easy chair reading his latest copy of *Analog*, the science-fiction magazine. I do not see lines, shadows, edges, colors, shapes. I see the whole, unified image of my dad. He turns a page. I see a seamless moving image of his hand reaching out and flipping the page.

Neuroscientists refer to this as the "binding problem." And it is a serious scientific question. One suggestion has been that the brain binds the different parts of an image together in time rather than space. That is, the brain uses a kind of timing mechanism to coordinate the simultaneous firing of all the neurons and neural networks in the different parts of the brain that analyze an image. Much of the experimental work exploring this possibility has been done with cats and monkeys. But since no one has ever been able to find a cat or a monkey suffering from a problem with binding features together, it's been hard to confirm with confidence these kinds of hypotheses.

Consider E.H., whom we met a little earlier. One of the consequences of her stroke is directly related to the binding problem. After her stroke, E.H. was found to suffer from a condition called face agnosia. Agnosia is the loss of comprehension of some sensation—visual, auditory, tactile, whatever—without any loss of sensory input. Another name for agnosia is "mind blindness." Face agnosia is the loss of the ability to recognize human faces, even though a person's visual perception and other senses remained mechanically functional. In E.H.'s case, she could no longer recognize the faces of her husband, daughter, relatives, or friends. She couldn't recognize her own face in a mirror, though she knew intellectually that it was hers. However, she could still recognize people by their voices. If she were sitting it a room facing away from the door and her husband came in and started talking, she knew immediately that it was he.

Most of us bind all these sensory perceptions together into a seamless whole. This is a complete and seemingly instantaneous gestalt experience that we can at once identify as our father, our mother, our wife or husband, a friend or neighbor; our pet cat; a pepperoni-and-mushroom pizza; a telephone. The point is, our brain appears to bind together many different bits and pieces of each such object, person, place, thing. For E.H., that seemingly seamless linkage has been broken.

ANNE TRIESMAN, a member of the Department of Psychology at Harvard University, has offered a possible solution to the binding problem. Triesman and her associates think that the human brain needs to pay close attention to the spatial locations of an object in order to bind its features together into a holistic impression. That is, the where network in the brain would play a vital role in feature binding. This is the kind of hypothesis that can be tested fairly easily with humans. One could, for example, disrupt a person's attention to an object's location in space, or one could give a human volunteer inaccurate spatial data about the object.

Exactly these kinds of tests have indeed been done with humans for many years. Triesman was doing this kind of work back in 1982; other, similar experiments date back to 1931. The typical experiment of this type is quite simple, and the results are dramatic. Suppose you, the researcher, present a human volunteer with brief glimpses of colored letters flashed on a screen. You also flash a number on the screen at the same time as the colored letter. You ask the subject to identify the number. If the "spatial location" hypothesis for feature binding is correct, this kind of confusing display should overload the "attentional network" of the person's brain. That is, the parts of the brain that are paying attention to the number's different features will get confused by the simultaneous display of a colored letter right next to the number. The result will be what psychologists call an *illusory conjunction*, or IC.

In fact, that's just what happens in these kinds of experiments. A person who is shown a blue X and a red 4, for example, will confidently reply that she has seen a red X and a blue 4. However, the normally functioning human brain is incredibly good at binding features together into seamless, unified images. In lab experiments, ICs occur only when the subjects undergo massive demands on their brains' attentional systems, *and* the displays they're looking at appear very briefly. "Briefly" is usually around 200 milliseconds. Under these kinds of severe conditions, a person will suffer illusory conjunctions. So this problem is almost never seen outside the laboratory.

And then there's the person known as R.M.

R.M. is a man in his late fifties who has suffered significant damage to his brain. First in June 1991 and again in March 1992, several blood vessels in R.M.'s brain became blocked. This caused several parts of his brain to be deprived of blood, and the neural tissue died. The damaged areas are in both the left and right cerebral hemispheres, in nearly identical parts of the parietal and occipital lobes. The parietal lobes stretch from the top of the brain toward the back, and the occipital lobe lies behind the parietal lobes at the very back of the brain. R.M.'s frontal lobes and temporal lobes remain undamaged and appear to function normally.

Researchers used magnetic resonance imaging (MRI) to take a set of images of R.M.'s brain. Those MRI images dramatically reveal the extent of the damage he has suffered. R.M.'s vision is normal—better than normal, in fact, since the visual acuity in both eyes tests at 20/15. He has normal color vision and normal sensitivity to contrast in light and dark parts of an image. The visual fields for both his eyes are almost completely normal.

Some people who suffer damage to one side of the brain will have problems paying attention to objects in the opposite field of vision. They will make more illusory conjunctions with objects appearing in that opposite field of vision than with those appearing in the same-side field of vision. R.M. does not appear to have any such problem with attention for the left or right visual field. Tests of his vision in 1994 also revealed that he could accurately judge if an object was moving toward or away from him. But R.M. does have very serious problems identifying *where objects are located*. Neurological tests done shortly after his strokes showed that R.M. even had a hard time telling if more than one object was present in a natural scene. I have eight trees in my backyard. When I look out the kitchen window onto that scene, I see eight trees. R.M., however, would be unable to tell that there was more than one tree.°

Stacia R. Friedman-Hill, then a graduate student at the University of California at Davis, along with Treisman and Lynn Robertson (also at U.C. Davis), decided to do some tests of R.M.'s feature binding abilities (Fig. 7.4). In their first set of tests (all done with R.M.'s permission, of course) Friedman-Hill and her colleagues had R.M. look at displays containing two colored letters. R.M.'s job was to tell them the name and color of the first letter he saw. In each trial, R.M. looked at two letters presented simultaneously. Each display consisted of a two-letter combination of red, yellow, and blue O's, T's, and X's. The shapes would flash onto the computer screen and remain there for half a second, three seconds, or ten seconds. R.M. looked at many different combinations of these letters. During one session, for example, he willingly underwent 104 different trials.

Each display of a two-letter combination could result in several different errors. For a display of a red T and a blue X, for example, he could report seeing a blue T and a red X (an IC error). He might also report seeing a yellow T or X or an O of some color. These are "intrusion errors," meaning they are "intrusions" of an object or color that was never present in the first place. Intrusion errors gave the researchers an estimate of the proportion of guesses R.M. might be making. They

---

°This is a medical condition known as Balint syndrome.

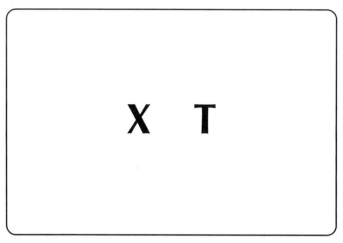

FIG. 7.4.   An example of R.M.'s first test for visual feature
binding. "What is the name and color of the first letter you
see on the screen?"

would also indicate problems with identifying the actual shapes of the
objects he was looking at. In fact, R.M. had few problems of this kind;
his intrusion error rate was less than 3 percent.

But he did have serious problems with illusory conjunctions. His IC
rate was 13 percent. This was true even when he had as long as ten seconds to look at the display of two letters. It was true even when he gave
the display his undivided attention.

Friedman-Hill and her colleagues then carried out another experiment with R.M. (Fig. 7.5). In this one, he looked at displays of two elementary geometrical shapes and was asked to tell which was the larger
of the two. The shapes included black diamonds, squares, and plus signs
in five different sizes. In one test sequence, a pair of shapes would be
simultaneously flashed onto a computer screen for R.M. to see and
remain on the screen for about three seconds. In another sequence, the
researchers would display each object in sequence in the middle of the
screen for about eight-tenths of a second.

Even though he had twice as much time to look at the images presented simultaneously as those presented in sequence, R.M. made significantly more mistakes discriminating among the former than the
latter. This pattern is exactly the opposite of that found in normal people who take this kind of test. That is, people with no neurological prob-

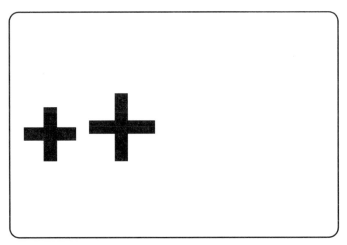

Fig. 7.5.   An example of R.M.'s second test for visual feature binding. Which plus sign is the taller? The one on the left or the one on the right?

lems do consistently better with the simultaneously presented images than with those they see in sequence. Friedman-Hill thinks that R.M.'s error pattern shows he can effectively compare two objects that appear in the same place at different times and tell which is larger than the other. But he can't compare two objects appearing at the same time and close to each other in space. It's not simply a problem with combining features to form an integrated object. This has to do with R.M.'s inability to use spatial location to visualize differences between two objects.

It was also clear to the researchers that R.M.'s mistakes were not simply failures of size discrimination. If that were the case, he would have made more errors when the size difference between the two objects was smaller. But the percentage of errors was nearly the same, no matter what the difference in size.

Finally, the researchers tested R.M.'s ability to judge the location of an object shown on a computer screen. In one series of tests, they showed him a letter X appearing either in one of five locations along a horizontal line through the middle of the screen or in one of five spots along a vertical line. R.M. was to tell them if the X was either to the left, right, or at the center of the screen or above, below, or at the center. In a second set of tests, they showed R.M. an X sitting next to an O (Fig. 7.6). He was to ignore the O and just report the location of the X on the

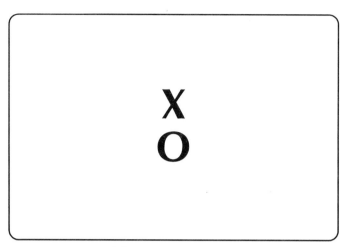

Fig. 7.6.   R.M.'s ability to judge location.
Where is the X in relation to the O?

computer screen. Finally, the researchers asked R.M. to tell them the location of the X relative to the O. In all these tests R.M. was looking at white letters on a black screen.

R.M. did not do very well. He averaged only 70 percent correct overall. While this is better than pure chance, it is actually a very low success rate for such an elementary set of tasks. And in the final set of tests, judging the location of the X relative to the O, he did no better than chance. R.M. was simply unable to tell if one object was to the left or right of the other.

R.M. can recognize letters; he knows the difference between left and right. But the damage to his parietal and occipital lobes has left his brain incapable of properly binding together the colors *and* the shapes of two or more objects at once. We need all that information—shape, color, motion, size, shading, texture, lines—to correctly identify an object, whether it is a red X or our father's face. R.M. has lost an important part of his spatial binding ability, and with it he has lost an essential part of his ability to see.

Yet out of his tragedy we are learning a little more about how the brain's many different subsystems work together to create the visual world in which we live.

CHAPTER 8

MEMORY AND LEARNING

E. M. FORSTER once said that "unless we remember we cannot understand." If true, what are we to make of my father's memory? He can't remember his children's exact birth dates. This may be because he has seven children; that's a lot of birthdays to remember. So he keeps a piece of paper in his wallet on which is written all our birth dates. Is it August? Peter and Ed have birthdays in August—but when? He checks the list and sees "8/9 Peter" and "8/17 Ed." If it's close enough to those dates, he and my mother will buy birthday cards and mail them. And then Dad forgets their birth dates until the next time.

However, he has no difficulty telling you how many picas there are in an inch ("Six," he says in an instant reply to my question) or how many points in a pica. ("Twelve.") Of course, my dad is a retired newspaper printer. He started working in his high school print shop in 1939 and didn't fully retire from his job at the Ventura County (Calif.) *Star Free-Press* until 1990. That's fifty-one years in the printing business, and he still knows points and picas as well as most of us know how to add two plus two.

CATEGORIES OF MEMORIES

Memory has long been one of the great mysteries of the human mind. Somehow the brain is able to take the constant influx of perceptual information and store it. What's more, much of that information is stored in way that is easily accessible, even after a lifetime, while the rest of it is soon discarded. In recent years brain researchers have confirmed that these two kinds of memory are handled by very different parts of the brain. They are not different versions of one another. The revolution in brain-imaging technology has even made it possible to see the brain's memory areas in action.

What we call memory is simply the storage and retrieval of information by the brain. Without memory, learning would be impossible. But memory is much more than recalling multiplication tables or that day in the park with your wife more than forty years ago. In fact, memory in all its forms is essential to survival. The nervous systems of all living creatures, from amoebas to antelopes, must store and recall both motor-skill memories and responses to environmental dangers. The ability to walk or run, to chew food and eliminate wastes, to avoid a cliff or run from the smell of a predator—these routine functions are all made possible by forms of memory.

Researchers sometimes speak of two general types of memory: *motor-skill memory* and *factual memory*. The ability to memorize motor skills, such as riding a bicycle or even walking, is a form of motor-skill memory. This kind of memory makes possible many routine functions without the need of much, if any, conscious thought. We all know that our first attempts at riding a bicycle involved great concentration and several spills. Our father or mother would trot along beside us, offering words of encouragement and the occasional steadying hand on the handlebars. Eventually, we somehow got the hang of it. Wobbly at first, we made our first triumphant trips along the sidewalk or in the driveway without a fall. Within a few months we were hopping on our little bike and pedaling off without a second thought. Motor-skill memory had taken over.

Recalling a telephone number, the plot of a book, or the name of your first boyfriend are all examples of factual memory. When my father first started working in the printing shop at Lynwood High School in 1939, he probably didn't know a pica from a point. A "cheat sheet" may have helped him at first. But it wasn't long before he had memorized the numerical conversions. Twelve points to a pica, about six picas to an inch—so a 48-point headline font is two-thirds of an inch tall. More than fifty years later, he recalls the conversions without the slightest hesitation. That's factual memory at work.

Another and more common way of categorizing memory is by its length or duration. *Immediate memory* is the ability to retain information long enough to perform tasks and maintain a train of thought.

Working memory (which used to be called short-term memory) is the ability to retain and recall data for more than a few minutes. It effectively functions as a bridge between new information and long-term memory. *Long-term memory* stores and retrieves information for anything from a few months to as long as a lifetime. The vagaries of my father's memory are examples of working memory and long-term memory. His ability to instantly recall that 12 points equal one pica is an example of long-term memory. His ability to recall his children's birth dates for only short periods of time is an example of working memory.

An electrical phenomenon called *long-term potentiation* (LTP) seems to be involved in long-term memory. We all have had what could be called intense learning experiences. One example from my own life that comes immediately to mind (to memory?) was my childhood realization that a Mobius strip has just one side. (Take a long, thin strip of paper by its two ends. Twist one of the ends over and then tape the two ends together. Now take a pencil and begin drawing a line on one side of the strip. Before long you'll see that the line you're drawing goes completely around the strip, on "both sides." Because there aren't two sides, but just one.) Spontaneous bursts of high-frequency electrical stimulation in the brain cause neurons to become more responsive. This is long-term potentiation, and it is involved in intense learning experiences. LTP might also explain the feelings of excitement and curiosity (*"One side!* Just *one* side! Wow!"*) that often accompany an intense learning experience.

The brain's limbic system also plays an important role in the processing of memories. And as we'll see in chapter 9, this region of the brain is Emotion Central. So it is not surprising that emotions affect memories. When the body undergoes emotional or physical stress, it produces steroid hormones. Since these chemicals increase alertness, a strong emotion, such as fear or grief, can imprint an experience indelibly on the memory. We all know that experience of sharpened awareness. Suppose, for example, we are suddenly in the middle of an auto accident on the freeway. Time seems to slow down; we see the oncoming car with remarkable clarity, along with the terrified face of the driver. Years later we can vividly recall that moment. Post-traumatic stress disorder (PTSD) is another very good example of the effects of strong emotion on memory. The intense memory flashbacks associated with PTSD are the result of the association of a strong emotion, such as fear with a particular event. Then there's the other side of the emotional coin. Prolonged stress can have just the opposite effect. It can interfere with memory storage. It is not uncommon for survivors of prolonged childhood sexual abuse, for example, to have huge gaps in their childhood memories. The prolonged emotional and physical stress of the abuse may have interfered with either the storage of the memories or the person's ability to retrieve them. Sometimes the memories do return, and the person then begins suffering the effects of PTSD. However, memory is also a tricky thing. Researchers like Dr. Elizabeth Loftus of the University of Washington have provided compelling evidence that it is possible to construct "false memories." These are memories of events that never happened. Again, intense emotions can play a role in the development of false memories. So can the efforts of a highly persuasive person who is—deliberately or not—trying to implant the memories.

Of course, we all have gaps in our memory, especially those from childhood. Sometimes such gaps are created by the mind in an attempt to avoid extreme psychological trauma. Most people with missing pieces of childhood memories, though, have not suffered such traumas. Their gaps probably have a more prosaic and commonplace cause, having to do with the way the brain creates and stores memory. The brain first stores new information in working memory. If this information—whatever it is, from multiplication tables to a sensory perception, like the shape of a hawk—is refreshed and reinforced often enough, it moves into long-term memory. Generally, information that is learned over an extended period of time is better remembered.

When I ask my father how many points there are in a pica, he will immediately answer, "Twelve." This long-term memory has been reinforced by more than fifty years as a printer. Every working day, my father dealt with points and picas, type sizes, and column inches. Just as most of us can quickly answer the question "What is five times four?" my dad can tell you about picas and point sizes. Ask him, however, to name my phone number and he will draw a blank. He'll look it up in his personal phone book and then remember it long enough to dial us up. But then he will forget it again, for it is no longer important. The phone number gets stored in his working memory until he is finished with it, and then it disappears.

If I ask my mother about the summer cabin she and her family would stay in during her childhood in Hungary, she can give me many details. She remembers its location, size, and shape ("Actually," she confides with a laugh, "it was just a remodeled chicken coop!") and the emotions she felt as a child when she stayed there. That's a childhood memory that has stayed in her brain's long-term-memory storage areas. Were I to ask her what meal her mother served on a particular date in 1935, however, my mother would have no idea. Nor does she have many clear memories of her school days in Budapest. These are memories that have simply disappeared. Never reinforced by recall or some strong emotional association, they have long departed.

Memory is most likely stored in two ways. The first involves a correlation of activity between neurons, such as the synchronous firing of many neurons or some kind of oscillating neuronal circuit. No one really knows how long information can be stored in the brain in this fashion. Some mathematicians believe it depends on the size of the network of neurons involved. Theoretically, they claim, the storage could be infinite—or at least as long as one lives.

The second mechanism has been studied in much more detail. This method involves storing information within the synapses by adjusting their strength. As we already know, the synapse is the tiny gap that exists between the end of one neuron and the membrane of another. Usually it's the gap between the tip of one neuron's axon and the surface of another neuron's dendrite or main cell body. Increasing the amount of neurotransmitter chemical released from the presynaptic terminal or increasing the postsynaptic response to a given amount of neurotransmitter—or both—would create changes in the strength of the synaptic response.

We can recover information stored in memory in several ways. Retrieving or reproducing learned material is called memory *recall*, or *retrieval*. *Recognition* is more limited, being simply the ability to identify something we have encountered before. An essay question seeking information about the origins of World War II tests a person's recall. A multiple-choice question about the date of the Pearl Harbor bombing tests a person's recognition. If I recognize a person's face but cannot recall her name, I have good recognition but bad recall. Often we may think we have forgotten some piece of information when we really have not. One example of this is with second languages. People who learn a second language as infants but never use it later on will as adults have a much easier time relearning that language than will people who never were exposed to the language in the first place. It thus appears that we do retain some memories even though we are no longer conscious of them.

Forgetting usually takes place when a memory is not used or activated for a period of time. And, of course, forgetting does serve several important functions. We can get rid of information that is no longer useful. Forgetting also allow us to orient ourselves to the present.

Forgetting is a normal process, but some forms of forgetting are far from normal. Head injuries can cause losses of memory known as *amnesia*. Several forms of amnesia exist. In *retrograde amnesia* a person cannot recall memories formed prior to the injury or trauma. Very severe head injuries can cause *anterograde amnesia,* in which *new* memories cannot be stored. *Traumatic automatism* is a form of amnesia in which a person functions normally but afterward remembers nothing. Amnesia can also be caused by organic disease. Korsakoff's syndrome can cause amnesia so severe that the person's brain cannot store new information anywhere but in immediate memory. With no working or long-term memory, these people live in an eternal present. Encephalitis can cause a similar type of amnesia. Brain surgery commonly causes some problems with memory. The person's memory will often return, but sometimes it will take years.

Sometimes a person will lose his or her memory without any known injury or disease. This is called *psychogenic amnesia*. Hypnosis can induce this kind of amnesia, in which events occurring during the hypnotic trance are forgotten. The psychological state known as *dissociation* (sometimes called hysterical amnesia) is one in which a specific memory cannot be recalled except under hypnosis or in dreams. Dissociation is frequently a psychological reaction to highly traumatic events in a person's life.

Some kinds of memory errors aren't quite extensive enough to be called amnesia. Memory experts call such errors *paramnesia*. *Confabulation* refers to the retrieval of false memories resulting from organic brain disease. A person suffering from confabulation will often report in great detail events that never occurred, apparently with no awareness that the memories are false. *Déjà vu* (from the French, meaning "already seen") is the sensation that a new event has happened to us before. Finally, we sometimes experience simple memory "deceptions" when we remember a dream, fantasy, or hallucination as a real event.

At the other end of the scale is *hyperamnesia*, a highly strengthened or accurate memory. One example of hyperamnesia is photographic memory, in which a person is able to store information in highly detailed and vivid terms.

YIN AND YANG

Without memory there is no such thing as true learning. And vice versa. Learning and memory go together like two dancers in a pas de deux. They are each other's yin and yang.

Definitions of "learning" abound; the study of its nature and processes has been a growth industry for centuries. Many scientists define it as the organization of behavior based on experience. All learning involves an interplay among the brain, the nervous system, and the environment. For it is nothing more or less than the process of acquiring skills, information, and knowledge. We do this by processing, categorizing, storing, and reusing information that comes to us through our senses. So memory is an integral part of the learning process; without it there would be no information to be stored and retrieved.

Learning affects an individual's behavior in a number of ways. One of the most obvious is the acquiring of a skill. If a person learns to tie shoelaces, ride a bicycle, or swim, that skill will remain with him or her and will be improved by practice. Other skills, like playing the violin° or programming a computer, are more difficult to acquire and will be virtually lost if they are not practiced frequently. Skills like cooking or driving a car may be partially lost through disuse but may be regained fairly easily.

An important feature of learning is known as concept formation, the ability to form concepts or ideas. An aspect of this type of learning is the ability to classify perceived objects by their similarities and differences. Consider, for instance, a boy walking down a street to the corner mailbox. He notices that the leaves on all the trees are virtually identical in shape. On his way back, he notices that the leaves on the other side of the street are all of a different shape. Based on these two sets of visual perceptions, he is able even without knowing botany to make a simple classification based on similarities and differences. Later, he learns that all the trees on one side are oaks, while those on the other side are maples. He is thereby able to give a name to the classifications he has already made by himself.

This ability to conceptualize, to form ideas, is necessary for higher levels of learning. A girl who is studying geometry must learn to perceive

---

°Which my father learned in high school and has never done since returning from World War II.

the differences among a variety of shapes: circles, triangles, and squares and other rectangles as well as the different shapes of the conic sections. The perceived differences will give her the idea, for instance, of a triangle. Triangles all share certain specific features that distinguish them from other shapes.

Ideas, as simple classifications and distinctions, are of limited value unless they are aided by training. An untrained ear may perceive three different pieces of dance music and only know that they are different. The trained musician will know that the first is a waltz, the second a samba, and the third a mazurka. It is by training and by naming that ideas get content whereby they can be shared. Animals other than human beings can perceive and remember differences in shapes, sounds, and smells. But they do not give names to the ideas they get; nor do they build upon their ideas over the passage of time. For humans, being able to name things and share ideas makes possible complex language and complex teaching systems. These are the basis of the human ability to exercise collective judgment, solve complex problems, and build on past learning.

THEORIES OF LEARNING

The more researchers have learned about the brain and nervous system and how they work, the more insights they have gained into the nature of learning. However, most of our understanding of the learning process has come from studying animals in both the laboratory and their natural habitats. In these studies, scientists define learning as some specific and permanent change in an animal's behavior that accompanies experience. Other factors are controlled for so that the researchers can isolate the specific environmental experience and the specific change in behavior that results. This makes it possible to measure behaviors and thus have some kind of numerical and repeatable measurements of the learning process.

From these kinds of experiments and observations, researchers have been able to identify several different types of learning. "Learning by association" is a good example. A young child touches a hot electrical coil on the kitchen stove and burns himself. He quickly associates touching the stove with pain. That's a form of learning by association called "stimulus-response," or S-R association. Conditioning is a form of learning by association that involves S-R. The classic example is the work of Ivan Pavlov, the Russian physiologist. In 1889, Pavlov first showed that a dog's nervous system mediates the stimulus that causes the animal's stomach and digestive system to secrete digestive juices. Thirteen years later, he formulated his theory of learning by conditioning. In his most famous experiment, Pavlov would ring a bell at the same time he gave food to a dog. Soon the dog would learn to salivate at the sound of the bell alone. The phrase "Pavlov's dogs" came to symbolize a mindless response to a particular stimulus. In fact, his dogs revealed the nature of a particularly basic kind of learning, one which all of us use.

Pavlov's experiments used positive reinforcement (the food) to establish S-R learning. Negative reinforcement can also create S-R learning. Example: If the house gets too hot for comfort in the wintertime, we go to the thermostat and turn down the heat. Still another kind of S-R learning uses punishment. The response decreases because it is followed by an unpleasant event. An infant cries because he wants to be picked up. The exasperated mother yells at the child each time he cries. The infant quickly learns to cry less frequently, not at all, or at least quietly in order to avoid the unpleasantness.

When any animal (including a human) links a certain event or signal with a specific condition, then that animal will soon develop an automatic response simply to the signal or event alone, whether or not the original condition is still in force. We all have such automatic learned responses. The unique, high-pitched buzzing sound that signals the imminent landing of a mosquito will automatically cause me to frantically wave my hands around. I can be almost asleep and that buzzing mosquito sound will trigger a flurry of arm waving and body slapping. Most people who live in towns or cities will automatically jump at the sudden sound of a nearby car horn; it doesn't matter if a car is actually nearby or not. Phobias are other examples of this kind of conditioning. An unreasoning fear of water (hydrophobia), terror at the sight of a spider (arachnophobia), the irrational inability to leave one's house and venture outside (a form of agoraphobia, or fear of open spaces)—these and other phobias may well have been formed by the initial association of something otherwise harmless with some threatening or dangerous stimulus.

Another form of learning, one with which most of us are quite familiar, is cognitive learning. Some researchers think that learning takes place through the organization of perceptions in ways that are useful. The German-American psychologist Wolfgang Kohler once showed that chimpanzees fit several sticks together in a makeshift pole to obtain food that was otherwise out of reach. This kind of behavior suggests a sudden understanding of how to solve the problem rather than aimless efforts of trial and error that finally stumble onto success. This is an example of the cognition theory of learning—learning by perceiving and using insight or knowledge.

For many years two separate schools of learning prevailed. One was the associationist emphasis on stimulus-response and trial and error. The other was the cognitive emphasis on reasoning and problem solving. Today most psychologists and learning theorists are convinced that people use both kinds of learning tactics. Kohler and other researchers have provided plenty of evidence that chimpanzees also use both cognition and trial and error to learn. How many species learn by cognition? It's a good question; and no one really knows the answer.

THE HIPPOCAMPUS REVEALED

Until fairly recently, in fact, there were few answers available about how the brain learns, how it stores what it learns as memories, and how it retrieves those memories. It is only in the last couple of decades that brain researchers have finally put to rest the long-held assumption that some specific area or areas were the repositories of memories. We now know that, like sensory perceptions, the brain stores learning and memory in many different areas at once. Those areas are connected by the interweaving of neurons and neural networks in ways that are still only partly understood.

One part of the brain that has long been suspected of playing an important role in memory is the hippocampus. The hippocampus is part of the brain's limbic system, a cluster of tiny ovoids and loops lying deep within the brain. The limbic system is part of the cerebrum, the part of the brain that sits atop the brain stem. The cortex is the visible, convoluted layer of nerve tissue sitting on top of the cerebrum. The hippocampus itself consists of two S-shaped loops of neural tissue, each wrapped around the left and right thalamus. In 1991, Marcus Raichle and his colleague Larry Squire of the University of California at San Diego confirmed that different parts of the brain perform different types of memory tasks. They also found the first unambiguous evidence that the hippocampus plays a major role in memory.

Squire and Raichle had eighteen volunteers perform several word-completion tasks, and they scanned their brains using positron-emission tomography (PET) as they did so. In one task, their subjects were to provide the researchers with the first word that came to their minds. In another task, the volunteers first looked over a list of words and were later asked to complete a word fragment by remembering a word from that list. For example, a person might be given the word fragment "mot" and would remember the word "motor" from the list. When they carried out this kind of memory task, the PET scans showed the right side of their hippocampus becoming very active. When the volunteers simply named the first word that came to their mind, however, neither side of the hippocampus became particularly active.

This particular discovery was somewhat surprising. As we'll see in more detail in chapter 10, most neuroscientists believe that this kind of verbal processing takes place in the brain's left hemisphere. But the PET scans were quite clear. Even though it involves verbal memories, when this kind of memory work is taking place, the right side of the hippocampus plays a major role.

Another unexpected discovery ensued. The participants in the tests at times spontaneously remembered a word from the list without recalling that they had even seen it before. Psychologists call this phenomenon "priming." When it took place, the PET scans of the volunteers' brains showed that the primary visual cortex was playing a major memory role.

MEMORY TO THE LEFT AND RIGHT

Different brain-scanning experiments have shown that the brain coordinates the memories of events we personally experience—known as episodic memories—even though those memories are stored in different brain regions. In 1994, PET scans revealed preliminary evidence of a "laterality" to the storage and retrieval of episodic memories. That is, one hemisphere of the brain is active when these memories are being stored, and the other is active when they're being recalled.

Endel Tulving is a psychiatrist and professor at the University of Toronto. Born in 1927 in Estonia, Tulving left when he was seventeen, with World War II still raging and the Soviets bearing down. From 1945 to 1947 he worked for the American forces as a translator in Germany. But it would be twenty years before he was finally reunited with his parents.

He currently resides in Toronto, Canada, where he has worked since the early 1950s at the University of Toronto. Though semiretired, he maintains an office at the Rotman Research Institute in Toronto and continues his research on memory.

"Cognitive psychologists study the human mind," Tulving has said. "They ask, 'How do we know anything?' 'What is a memory?' " He has made the study of the brain's memory networks his life's work.

Tulving has long held the theory that memory has two separate and distinct parts. The first is the process by which the brain creates and stores memories. The second is the process of retrieving them. These are separate functions, he feels, that are governed by different parts of the brain.

As an example of this, Tulving has written of a classroom experiment he has conducted with his students. He will have the students sit quietly and listen as he recites a few dozen words. When he has finished, he has them write down as many of the words as they can remember. Most of the students recall eight to ten of the words Tulving has recited. Once they're finished writing, he will pick up a student's paper and notice a word that did not get written down. He will ask, "Do you remember a color?" At once the student says, "Yellow," which in fact was one of the words Tulving had spoken earlier. "Do you recall a small animal?" "Cat," another student replies. He repeats this round of questioning with other students and other missed words. They soon understand his point: Just because we cannot remember a word doesn't mean it's not there.

Tulving has used PET scans in two different studies involving episodic memory. In the first, twelve men carefully studied two lists of common nouns. The men saw the lists on a computer screen as they lay in the PET scanner. After a twenty-minute pause, the men carried out two different memory tasks. As they did so, the researchers carried out PET scans on their working brains. In the first, they were asked to detect the presence or absence of the letter "a." For example, this list might include words like apple, berry, coffee, dragon, elephant, and so on. Asked to recall a word with an "a" in it, the volunteers would try to remember apple, dragon, or elephant. In the other task, the subjects categorized each noun as living or nonliving. The second list might have words like avenue, barber, chair, deer, elevator, and so on. Asked to recall nouns from the list that were living, volunteers would be trying to remember barber or deer rather than avenue or elevator.

Tulving and his colleagues found, first of all, that the men did a better job of remembering the words they analyzed by meaning (living or nonliving?) than the words analyzed by letters (an "a" or not?). Tulving also compared the PET images of the two cognitive tasks. This revealed a significant increase in activity in the brain's left inferior prefrontal cortex in the semantic task (living versus nonliving), as compared to the perceptual task. (Is there an "a" in the word or not?) This is part of the brain's outer layer that is behind the forehead and just in front of the left temple, hidden within (the medical meaning of "inferior") one of the cortex's ridges. Tulving believes that this part of the brain is actively involved in the storage of new verbal material, particularly when the new material is being interpreted in light of previous knowledge.

In Tulving's second study, another twelve men first listened to a tape-recorded list of rather unusual definitions for words. For example, the word "trampoline" was defined as "a form of recreation for the jumpy." The following day, the men underwent PET scans of their brains as they listened to a second tape recording. This one included both the word definitions they'd heard the day before and some new ones as well. The researchers then used computers to mathematically subtract the PET images made while the men first heard the new definitions (the "novel stimulus," as a psychiatrist would put it) from the scans made while they listened to the definitions they'd heard the previous day.

The result was a set of PET images showing brain activity in several regions, but not in the areas activated during the first tests. One of the active areas during this study of memory recall lay to the side and toward the rear of the right prefrontal cortex. Both parietal lobes, lying to the rear of the brain, were also active. So was a fold of tissue lying deep in the brain near the corpus callosum, that thick band of neurons that connects the brain's two hemispheres. Called the cingulate sulcus, this neural fold is close to the hippocampus, which we've already seen also plays an important role in memory.

Much of the brain activity that Tulving detected with the PET scans was taking place in the depths of cortical fissures, or sulci. The increases in blood flow detected by PET—and thus an increase in brain activity—Tulving thinks is evidence of a widely distributed neural network for the conscious retrieval of the memories of previous events. This network includes neuron clusters in the right prefrontal cortex and both parietal lobes. That much of this activity takes place in the brain's cortical fissures is also intriguing. Tulving theorizes that memory-related processes may require a high density of neurons and synaptic connections, a condition that exists in the deep folds of the cortex.

ALAN GEVINS AND MEMORY

While PET has occupied center stage in recent years in the study of the brain, memory, and learning, other imaging technologies are also being used with considerable success. One is the enhanced EEG technology developed by Alan Gevins at the EEG Systems Laboratory in San Francisco.

When I visited his office, Gevins talked about two studies in particular that dealt with working memory. One was reported in a scientific paper he published in 1993. In the study, five people hooked up to enhanced EEGs began by staring at a blank screen. They were waiting for a number to flash on the screen. During this time the EEG recorded their brain waves and thus provided a "control" for the rest of the test.

When the number flashed on the screen, each volunteer was supposed to move a finger in proportion to the number. After a short pause, another number would flash on the screen. Again a short pause, then another number would appear. Now came the interesting part of the test. Each volunteer was supposed to compare this latest number with the number from *two trials back*. This means that the subject had to remember the last two numbers seen in order to make the comparison. If the number was *not* the same as the one two trials back, the subject had to provide the finger response that he or she had used for that earlier number. The EEG recordings, said Gevins, reveal that "these neural networks for working memory are very rich and elaborated, while the control condition networks are very simple.

"This is an example of a complex network representing a simulation of two numbers," Gevins continued, "during a case of having to see more numbers and then respond to them. It's a very clear-cut situation. The subjects are staring at a blank screen. There's nothing else going on. The working-memory pattern only lasts a few hundred milliseconds—and then the stimulus comes on and there's a *different* pattern."

Another study by Gevins and his team also looked at working memory under conditions of mental fatigue. The subjects in this test, done in the late 1980s, were five air force test pilots from Edwards Air Force Base.* "These were guys who were trying really hard," said Gevins, even though they had been doing this memory task for six to eight hours. The

---

*Edwards is the air force's premier flight-testing facility and one of the two primary landing sites for the Space Shuttle.

basic finding of this study was that the brain's EEG patterns had started to change long before the pilots' mental fatigue became apparent in their behavior. In fact, the EEG patterns had changed a good two hours before their performance on the memory tests started getting less accurate. "They've been compensating," said Gevins, "and you can see a picture of that" with his enhanced EEG studies.

"The stimulus processing pattern doesn't change with time; it stays the same. After many hours the brain's extraction of the visual features isn't really different. But the process of holding the two numbers in the mind fatigues," Gevins explained. "The process that requires the mental concentration is fatiguing." And that degradation in working memory showed up in Gevins's enhanced EEG recordings long before the pilots themselves consciously knew about it.

PET AND LEARNING

Just as PET has played an important role in understanding memory, it is also helping brain scientists learn more about learning. One researcher who has provided some intriguing PET images of the brain at work as it learns is Richard J. Haier. Haier is a neuropsychologist at the University of California at Irvine. He and his colleagues have been using PET to measure the rate at which the brain uses glucose. As we saw in chapter 4, this form of sugar is the brain's main fuel. By labeling glucose molecules with tiny amounts of radioactive atoms, such as oxygen, researchers like Haier can track the brain's activity as it uses the glucose. The more active the neurons are, the more glucose they need to consume to keep their energy levels up. The more glucose they use, the greater is the amount of positron radiation coming from their part of the brain. The result: color-coded computer images of those parts of the brain that are working hard or hardly working.

Many researchers have long believed that the harder the brain works, the more it learns and the smarter a person is. Think of this as the "Protestant-work-ethic-theory" of learning and intelligence. Until the advent of imaging technologies like PET, however, there had been no way to directly test this assumption. In a series of studies since the late 1980s, Haier has been doing just that.

What he has found flies in the face of the Protestant-work-ethic theory of learning and intelligence. His results are better explained by what might be called the "mellow-out theory" of intelligence and learning. In a 1988 study, Haier did PET scans of volunteers as they took a test of their abstract, nonverbal reasoning skills. The eight men with high scores all displayed *reduced* glucose metabolism, and thus lowered energy use, in the brain areas being used in the test. In 1992, Haier did PET scans of another eight men who daily practiced a computer game called Tetris. This game involves moving and rotating differently shaped two-dimensional colored blocks and then dropping them to the bottom of the screen to create solid rows of blocks. After one to two months of playing Tetris daily, the PET scans showed that all eight men had sharp drops in overall brain activity while they were playing the game. Moreover, the men who had previously scored the highest on a test of abstract reasoning were the ones with the least brain activity while playing Tetris.

These initial findings led Haier to hypothesize the "mellow" theory of intelligence and learning. That is, smart brains solve complex problems not by working harder and gobbling up glucose but by working *more efficiently* and conserving energy. A more recent study appears to confirm this hypothesis.

Haier worked with two groups of volunteers. The first group consisted of seventeen adults who were mildly developmentally disabled. Seven of the volunteers had Down syndrome; all scored between 50 and 70 on a standard IQ test. ("Normal" intelligence on the Stanford-Binet test is indicated by scores between 85 and 115.) None of the people in this group had any evidence of physiological brain damage or injury. The second group included eleven adults with above-average intelligence, according to the Stanford-Binet test; they all had scores of 115 or greater.

Each person in both groups carried out a simple attention task while their brains underwent PET scans. The test involved watching a series of numbers flash on a computer screen and pressing a button whenever a zero appeared. Haier then compared the PET scans of the first group with those from the second. The developmentally disabled people used about 20 percent more energy throughout their brains than did the people in the second group. Haier had thus confirmed the flip side of the coin. Not only is highly efficient energy use a hallmark of brains at the right end of the intelligence bell curve, where all the really smart people are; less efficient energy usage appears to be a hallmark of the brains at the other end of the intelligence bell curve.

LEARNING AND GENDER

One of the most controversial areas of learning theory centers on the question of gender differences. Do women learn differently than men? And if so, why? In particular, what differences exist between the brains of men and women, and how are such differences related to learning?

Richard Haier may have found at least one such difference, and its connection to learning is an intriguing one.

Mathematics is an area of intellectual endeavor in which men rather than women have long been assumed to naturally excel. In reality, the statistics related to this argument are a bit complex. On most standardized tests of mathematical ability, girls generally outperform boys throughout most of childhood. Only when children enter puberty and begin middle school, junior high school, or high school do boys begin to outperform girls in mathematical ability. Curiously (or perhaps not so curiously), this is about the same time that young girls in general begin losing interest in science.

Most of this change in mathematical "ability" for girls and young women is directly or indirectly attributable to environmental influences. Peer pressure, for example, is a powerful psychological influence on both boys and girls as they enter their teenage years. The pressure to conform, to not stand out, to be acceptable to those of your own gender and attractive to those of the opposite gender, can be pretty overwhelming. Consciously or unconsciously, girls entering puberty soon learn that "smart girls" are not attractive to boys. They learn that "standing out" as smarter than one's peers is a sure way to be ostracized. Girls who like math are geeky, and that's not an attractive characteristic.

Haier and his group did PET scans of forty-four college students—men and women—as they took a mathematical-reasoning test. Eleven of the men and eleven of the women had previously scored above 700 on the math portion of the Scholastic Aptitude Test. A score of 800 is the highest possible. The other twenty-two students had all scored in the average range on the SAT math test.

Haier's PET scans revealed that the high-SAT-score men had large increases in energy use and thus brain activity throughout their brains as they worked at the mathematical-reasoning test. But the men with the average SAT scores had much smaller increases in brain activity. On the other hand, the high-SAT-score women all showed significant *decreases* in brain activity as they did the mathematical test. The only part of their brains that showed increased activity on the PET scans was the caudate nucleus. A similar drop in brain activity as well as a smaller increase in blood flow to the caudate nucleus took place in the brains of the women who had had average SAT scores. The comma-shaped caudate nucleus, by the way, is one of the four structures that make up the basal ganglia, located deep in the forebrain. The basal ganglia have long been thought to play an important role in physical movements by relaying information from the cerebral cortex to the brain stem and cerebellum. The caudate nucleus produces the brain chemical dopamine, which plays a major role in much of the brain's activities. Until now, though, no one suspected that it had anything to do with mathematical ability. However, it appears from Haier's PET scans that the caudate nucleus is somehow involved in mathematical reasoning in both men and women.

Perhaps just as important is the other part of Haier's results. Brain efficiency versus brain activity may be important for some learning process but not others. In particular, Haier thinks these findings indicate that "brain capacity is more important for high math ability in males, and brain efficiency is more important for high math ability in females."

So what's going on here? Good question. A psychologist at Johns Hopkins University in Baltimore has offered a suggestion. Julian Stanley has pointed out an interesting aspect of math ability in adolescent boys and girls. In national studies of twelve-year-olds, the boys outnumber the girls almost three to one at the highest levels of math ability. However, among girls the scores rise dramatically for those who identify themselves as having strong aesthetic values, such as a passion for form and beauty. Meanwhile, more "practical" values—such as wanting to know how machines work—are strongest in those boys who score highest on math tests. Stanley thinks that these tests, along with Haier's PET scans, suggest an actual difference in cerebral organization for certain kinds of learning tasks. In some areas, such as mathematical ability, there may be some overlapping between men and women.

USE IT OR LOSE IT

We continue to learn all of our lives. Learning of some kind doesn't stop until we die. For most of us, however, "learning" in this sense is the unconscious or nonconscious kind. We learn to avoid some novel and unpleasant stimulus. We learn to enjoy a new food. We learn what it feels like when a parent dies. If we read books, we learn a few new words as the years go by. Sadly, most of us most of the time don't do much new *conscious* learning. As we grow older, reach retirement, and head into our sixties and seventies, we rarely make the effort to expand our intellectual horizons. Blame it on television, blame it on a bad diet, blame it on the Republicans (or the Democrats); blame it on whatever or whomever you wish. The truth is, most of us are too lazy or too psychologically "asleep" to bother.

We should. For the last ten years or more, evidence has been mounting that the brain is like an intellectual muscle. The more we use it, the better it gets at doing what it does. Anecdotal evidence (which isn't scientific but certainly can count for something) suggests that elderly people who actively engage in new intellectual pursuits are generally happier, healthier, and live longer. By contrast, one research study done in the early 1990s suggests just the opposite for inactive but otherwise normal older people.

John Meyer, a neurologist at Baylor College of Medicine in Houston, followed ninety-four men and women who were about sixty-five years old at the beginning of the study. One-third of this group continued to work at regular jobs. A second third of the group was retired but still active. Some gardened, some bicycled regularly, and so on. The rest of the group was pretty much inactive. They stayed home and watched TV. Four years after the first set of tests, the people in the inactive group scored significantly lower on a battery of psychological tests than they had at the beginning. Just as important was that the blood flow in their brains had also dropped.

Haier's work with PET scans and learning suggests that some types of learning in humans require the brain to work harder, while other kinds of learning activities require it to work "smarter" or more efficiently. Meanwhile, a wealth of data from animal experiments has revealed that learning increases the number of synaptic connections among the animal's brain cells. Researchers have long known this is the case in human infants and young children, and we looked at that in some detail in chapter 4. No firm evidence yet exists that the same kind of synaptic growth takes place in the brains of human adults—of any age— as they learn. It's true, as one skeptical neuroscientist has said, that you can't always extrapolate the results from rats to humans. However, the anecdotal evidence for the "use it or lose it" theory of learning into old age is certainly intriguing.

Even if most brain scientists haven't yet found the hard evidence for this in their PET scans and MRI images, many are still putting it into practice. One noted neuroscientist in his sixties plays trombone and leads a jazz band. Another builds rock walls and does landscape painting. Still another plays mental games and practices learning new languages. Gene Cohen, who has worked for the National Institute on Aging, believes that intellectual activity is an important brain stimulus that actually makes neurons larger and healthier. Elderly people, he has said, who keep mentally active are generally more able to retain their intellectual sharpness as they grow older. They will also be happier than their more inactive friends and acquaintances.

It's good advice. No matter how old you are.

PART III

MAPPING THE MIND

The mind is an enchanting thing,
is an enchanted thing, like the glaze on a katydid-wing
    subdivided by sun
    till the nettings are legion.
—Marianne Moore, "The Mind Is an Enchanting Thing"

CHAPTER 9

THE EMOTIONAL BRAIN

IN THE SUMMER of 1989 I began experiencing panic attacks. I was forty years old, had gone through a divorce the previous year and the more recent breakup of an intense romantic relationship. My financial situation was shaky, and I was working hard on the manuscript that would later become my book *Mapping the Code: The Human Genome Project and the Choices of Modern Science*. However, I was also by all accounts in good physical health and was exercising more and eating better than I had in years. I had made new friends since my divorce and also reestablished a cautious but pleasant relationship with my former wife. So the onset of the panic attacks took me by complete surprise. They made no sense to me at all. I had not suffered from stage fright, for example, since grade school. I positively enjoyed standing in front of a crowd and delivering a lecture and then answering questions. For nearly a decade I had attended numerous science-fiction conventions as a professional writer of science fact, sitting on panels and often serving as the moderator.

Now, though, the mere thought of standing up in front of an audience made me sweat and shake. Actually doing it was often sheer terror. I was sure that at any moment I would collapse into unconsciousness or have some kind of seizure. The panic attacks occurred in other situations as well: driving across a freeway overpass, for example, or on a bridge that I had traversed uncounted times in the past, became a profoundly scary experience. While I had occasionally felt tinges of acrophobia, a fear of high places, I now found myself experiencing bouts of agoraphobia, the fear of open spaces. It all seemed completely absurd.

I *liked* open spaces—wide beaches stretching on for miles, a mountain meadow carpeted with wildflowers, Embarcadero Plaza in San Francisco. Now I was finding myself quaking in fear as I tried to cross the street.

After about six months the panic attacks began to subside in frequency. A year later, they seemed to occur only occasionally. But they continue to recur. Some, like the anxiety attacks before and during public-speaking situations, have never really relented. I have simply learned ways to endure until the irrational feeling of fear begins to fade.

About 15 percent of all Americans, some 27 million people, will suffer from an anxiety disorder such as panic attacks sometime in their lives. These disorders can be thought of as an overreaction of our normal "flight or fight" response to physical stress or danger. According to Stephen Dager, codirector of the University of Washington Center for Anxiety and Depression, these disorders are amenable to treatment. But most sufferers do not receive appropriate care. Most of us with anxiety disorders will seek relief from the physical symptoms, such as rapid heart rate, respiratory distress, or nausea, and may not be aware or want to admit that there are emotional causes for the symptoms.

"People worry about being labeled crackpots if they admit to overwhelming anxiety or fear," Dager has said. "But there is evidence that these symptoms are the result of healthy coping mechanisms gone awry. And worrying about them tends to exaggerate their effects."

There are several different types of anxiety disorders. The most common:

- Panic disorder is probably the best studied and understood of the anxiety disorders. It is characterized by repeated, unprovoked attacks of terror, accompanied by physical symptoms, including chest pain, heart palpitations, shortness of breath, dizziness, weakness, and sweating.
- Generalized-anxiety disorder (GAD) is "free-floating" anxiety or a constant unrealistic worry about two or more everyday occurrences which effect an individual's ability to complete daily activities. GAD is associated with physical anxiety symptoms, such as muscle aches, fatigue, difficulty sleeping, sweating, dizziness, and nausea.
- Phobia is a persistent, intense, and irrational fear associated with a particular object or situation that leads to avoidance of the object or situation.

- Social phobia is a persistent fear of one or more situations in which the person is exposed to possible scrutiny by others and fears that he or she may do something or act in a way that will be humiliating. Social phobias can also include extreme shyness.
- Obsessive-compulsive disorder (OCD) is characterized by repeated, intrusive, and unwanted thoughts (obsessions) that cause anxiety, often accompanied by ritualized behaviors (compulsions) that relieve the anxiety. Common obsessions include fear of dirt, germs, or contamination or fear of harming someone; common compulsions are excessive cleaning, counting, double-checking, and hoarding.
- Post-traumatic stress disorder (PTSD) is caused when someone experiences a severely distressing or traumatic event; individuals become so preoccupied with the experience that they are unable to lead a normal life.

So what exactly happened to me? How and why did these panic attacks begin? A therapist might point to the immense emotional and psychological stress I was under in 1988 and 1989 as a likely cause. I would be inclined to agree. However, emotional disturbances like my panic attacks must also have some physiological grounding in the brain. Neuroscientists have long known that certain brain structures create and control our most basic emotions, such as fear, rage, pleasure, and sexual desire. And we all know from personal experience that much of the time our emotions are not our masters. The jolt of fear we experience at, say, a sudden sonic boom from a high-flying jet plane will soon fade if we hear sonic booms several times a day, every day. Somehow, under many circumstances, our brains learn to either suppress or ignore emotional triggers. But how? And why are millions of us not able to suppress the emotional reactions that cause phobias, panic attacks and PTSD?

Even if it should make no difference in my ability to control or eliminate these pesky panic attacks, I'd certainly like to know what's going on behind the walls of my own skull. Now it is becoming possible to do so. Using time-tested experimental methods as well as the new suite of brain imagers, researchers are beginning to sketch out the brain's wiring diagram for emotions. In doing so, neuroscientists are going where generations of philosophers and psychologists have been either unwilling or unable to tread.

DEFINING EMOTIONS

Defining emotions is a lot like defining good art—or, for that matter, pornography. Ask a friend or coworker to define "emotion" and you'll likely get an answer like "Emotions are feelings" or "Oh, you know, fear or anger" or "Emotions are irrational impulses." Judy L. Lewis, the clinical supervisor for Community Mental Health in Washington State's Whatcom County, defines emotions as "a psychobiological response to changes in either our internal or external environment." Emotions are usually considered to be accompanied by a certain amount of internally or mentally experienced "excitement."

But that's not necessarily true. "There are plenty of clinical studies," Lewis notes, "clearly showing that every conscious thought we have is linked to some emotion. But for some people those emotions or feelings do not become conscious. That's why advertising can get away with a certain amount of subliminal persuasion." And because emotions are so intimately tied to thought, it may be misleading to refer to them as irrational.

Now ask your friend or coworker to name some emotions. Here you'll find little disagreement. We may not be able to define "emotion" clinically, as Lewis can, but we can certainly name them: acceptance, anger, anticipation, disgust, fear, grief, happiness, joy, sadness, surprise. Those are only a few emotions that come to people's minds and that arise in each of us at different times.

Any explanation for emotions must take into account three factors: what triggers the emotion, how the brain and mind respond, and how those responses in turn effect the way we internally experience the emotion. This is all complicated by the vague and at times contradictory vocabulary we use when talking about emotions. Because the word *emotion* itself has different meanings for different people, many scientists prefer to use the word *affect* (the pronunciation puts stress on the first syllable—AF-fect) to mean emotion. Other researchers think that affect should only be considered the part of an emotion we consciously experience, apart from unconscious responses or body responses. Thus, an affect is the same as a feeling. But the word *feeling* is also often used to refer to the sense of touch. Finally, a *mood* is an emotion that persists.

The conventional view of emotion in biology and psychology through the end of the nineteenth century was tied to the work done by Charles Darwin. The founder of modern evolutionary theory carried out studies of emotional expression in both humans and animals. This view held that emotional expressions depend not only on some previous emotional mental state but also on the evolutionary history of those emotional states and expressions. So some physical stimulus caused a mental state of fear as a response. That mental response in turn manifested itself in some sort of physical expression. In the case of a dog, for example, that physical response might be the cowering posture.

In the late nineteenth century two researchers, Carl Lange and William James, independently broke from this position. They essentially held that the perception of some stimulus directly causes a physical change in the body and that, as James wrote, "our feelings of the same changes as they occur *is* the emotion." In other words, for each specific emotional experience a particular pattern of body changes must exist. The problem with this theory was simple and far-reaching. No physical evidence could be found for these correspondences of emotion and specific somatic changes.

These deficiencies led a famous American physiologist to come up with a new theory of emotion. Walter Bradford Cannon was born in 1871, in Prairie du Chen, Wisconsin. It was the same year that Darwin's book *The Descent of Man* was published. Early in his career Cannon played a crucial role in the maturation of a then-still-new medical imaging technology. He developed a way for X rays to image the body's soft internal organs by using bismuth compounds.° Following World War I, Cannon proposed the medical theory of homeostasis, which states that the body tries to maintain a constant internal state.

Cannon's response to the James-Lange position on emotions was equally significant. He developed the *thalamic theory* of emotion. This was a neurophysiological position, as opposed to the James-Lange psychological stance, and it has had a profound influence on subsequent efforts to study and understand emotion and emotions.

The thalamic theory suggests that emotions are created by the neural stimulation of areas in the thalamus. The thalamus lies at the bottom of the forebrain† and consists of two egg-shaped masses of nerve cells lying at the base of the two cerebral hemispheres. The thalamus and

---

°Bismuth (its chemical abbreviation is Bi) is a white crystalline metal with a pinkish tinge. It has a low melting point (271.3° C). Because it's a metal, bismuth compounds used in liquids provide the opacity to make soft-tissue organs visible in X-ray images.

†Which, as you may recall, is the largest part of our brains and consists largely of the left and right cerebral hemispheres.

several other neural structures are part of what's collectively called the limbic system. It is nestled underneath the corpus callosum, that thick band of nerve fibers that connects the forebrain's two hemispheres.

According to Cannon's theory, the neural stimuli that travel to the thalamus and create emotions are normally suppressed or controlled by the neural activity of the cerebral cortex. Sometimes, though, a particularly strong stimulus will bypass the cortex's "emotional censors" and make it directly to the thalamus with no dilution in strength. Other emotions, called acquired emotions, depend on the brain's ability to recognize and remember certain kinds or classes of events that have some sort of emotional meaning. When some stimulus, external or mental, activates such a memory in the cortex, the emotional censors in the cortex are also activated. Neural signals from the activated thalamus in turn cause responses in both the peripheral nervous system and in the cortex. The signals sent to the peripheral nervous system are responsible for our physical responses to an emotion. The signals that go back to certain areas in the cortex create our subjective experience of that emotion.

When researchers removed the cortex from experimental animals, they found that the animals became hyperemotional. Their emotions would rage out of control. This would seem to be proof of the validity of Cannon's thalamic theory. But, as we noted earlier, the brain is never as simple as it first seems. When researchers then removed the thalamus from experimental animals, their hyperemotionality remained. These and other later studies eventually pointed to another brain structure as playing a major role in emotions: the hypothalamus.

The hypothalamus lies below and just forward of the connection between the two egg-shaped nuclei that make up the thalamus. The hypothalamus itself has several distinct substructures that have been linked to the regulation of the body's water balance and heat control. We now know from numerous animal and human studies that parts of the hypothalamus also play a role in regulating sex drive, hunger, aggressive behavior, and pleasure.

EMOTIONS AND ACTIVE BALANCE

When Walter Cannon first devised his homeostatic theory, he assumed that the balance of the body's internal systems and subsystems was a passive one. The autonomic nervous system, he asserted, was like a thermostat in a house, acting only when the temperature gets too hot or too

cool. Doctors and medical researchers now know that the body's autonomic and sympathetic nervous systems are much more active than this.
They both mobilize the body's internal systems for action and prepare
the organism to act upon the external environment.

Events that threaten a person's physical well-being, such as pain or
physical injury, will arouse the autonomic nervous system. Our more
sophisticated understanding of body homeostasis led researchers to
realize that other kinds of stressors will also trigger the autonomic nervous system. Any sudden or unexpected disruption of thought, action, or
perception will do the trick. We continually and unconsciously assume
that the world is fair, and then we get fired from our job for no dis-
cernible reason. We take the same bicycle route every day to the grocery
store and back, and one afternoon we come around the corner and find
the street blocked by massive earthmoving machines. The phone rings,
and we answer it, expecting still another telemarketing pitch; instead,
we hear the voice of our son in the navy, whom we haven't seen in a year:
"Dad, I've gotten leave, and I'm coming home to visit!"

These kinds of external stimuli, though not in the least bit threatening to our physical survival, will also trigger the autonomic nervous system. Once aroused, other actions take place. So emotional arousal
occurs in response to events of any kind that the organism finds important in some way. Events or stimuli that differ from expectations, from
past experiences and memories, from ingrained habitual patterns—
these, too, trigger responses in the brain and nervous system that we call
emotions. Which in turn suggests that emotions are not merely disrup-
tive or annoying intrusions into our otherwise normal and "rational"
lives. Emotions are adaptive responses as well. What is different is
important. The emotional experience marks and emphasizes its importance. Meanwhile, the autonomic nervous system's reaction and
response to these *different* events or stimuli make it possible for the person to adapt to the change, to change in response to the difference and
move onward.

THE COGNITIVE CONNECTION

Aristotle believed that emotions had roots that were partly physical and
partly mental. His suspicion turns out to have been close to the mark.
Today many researchers and theorists agree that any emotion begins
with the detection of something "different" about an event or other

stimulus. As we just saw, that "difference" does not simply have to be something that constitutes a physical threat. It can be anything that is new, different, or a disturbance in the normal flow of life.

Next comes a visceral reaction to the stimulus, triggered by the autonomic nervous system. This reaction is therefore outside the control of the person's conscious mind. The body enters a state of arousal. The person's heartbeat increases. The diaphragm's movements change, modifying the breathing of the lungs and thus pumping more oxygen into the blood. Certain hormones* stimulate the liver to release more sugar into the bloodstream. (Sugar is a great energy food.) The pupils of the eyes dilate, allowing as much light as possible to hit the retina and send visual data back into the brain. The muscles of the stomach and the intestines tighten up. If this state of physical arousal persists for some length of time, it essentially becomes a stressor. However, these arousal responses can also be small, almost unnoticed.

Much of the time, though, the person's conscious mind *does* take notice of the physical responses. How the conscious mind responds depends on the person's unique set of experiences and memories. What one person finds frightening another person may not. What you find to be erotic, she may find boring. I know several people who are utterly terrified at the sight of a snake, while I find them interesting to look at and almost enjoyable to touch.

So our cognitive abilities, our abilities to consciously evaluate and respond to stimuli based on our experiences and memories, play a vital role in our experience of emotions. Both positive and negative emotional states arise from the interaction of our nervous system's response to a "different" event and our individual cognitive responses to both the stimulus itself and to our body's response to it.

External stimuli aren't the only triggers of emotions. Memories can arouse emotions as powerful as any caused by an immediate experience. Sometimes that memory may be triggered by a physical stimuli. Whenever I hear the late-1950s rock ballad "Deep Purple Dream," I am immediately transported back to an autumn day when I was perhaps ten or eleven years old, lying on the living-room couch after school as the

---

*A hormone is a biological substance, usually a protein or a peptide, secreted by certain glands or nerve cells, which regulate the growth or function of some tissue or organ in a distant part of the body. For example, insulin is a hormone that controls how the body uses glucose sugar.

song played on the radio and *feeling* an almost indescribable complex of emotions that included sadness, sexual arousal, and what is best described as *yearning*. All it takes is the first few bars of that song and I'm gone. But even my mind alone can trigger this emotional response. I can be anywhere, and if I recall the tune from memory, the emotions flood back.

JOSEPH LEDOUX AND FEAR

One of the researchers exploring the biological territory of emotions and reason is Joseph LeDoux of New York University. LeDoux studies the neurological mechanisms of an emotion we have all experienced, one we know quite intimately: fear. He studies the fear mechanisms in animals, and his research reveals much about fear in humans and in human brains. On a practical level, his work will lead to new insights and possibly treatments for some of the most debilitating psychiatric disorders in humans. Anxiety, panic attacks, phobias, and PTSD all involve malfunctions of the brain's ability to control fear.

LeDoux and his colleagues have been tracing out the brain's fear pathways using experimental techniques that have been around for generations. He works with rats and focuses on a tiny structure deep in the brain called the amygdala. The amygdala is a tiny knot of brain cells that lies just underneath the thalamus. Like the thalamus, it is considered part of the small complex of neural structures at the bottom of the forebrain called the limbic system.

Researchers have known for years that the amygdala plays a crucial role in the creation of memories associated with emotions. If a rat's amygdala is damaged or destroyed, it will "forget" to be afraid. LeDoux's experiments have taken advantage of this to probe the connections throughout the rat brain that control how the animal appears to become used to a fear-causing stimulus. One particular series of experiments in the late 1980s and early 1990s produced incontrovertible evidence as to the way one area in the brain controls emotional memories originally created in the amygdala. These particular experiments began with a classic "Pavlov dog"–type of conditioning process. The researchers first administered mild electrical shocks to the rat's feet. At the same time, they piped a loud noise into the rat's cage. The rats quickly learned to associate the noise with the pain of the electrical shock. Soon the rats would show the physical reactions associated with a fear response just by hearing the noise. As time passed, though, the rats began to lose their fear of the sound. Either the amygdala was no longer producing the conditioned fear reaction, or some other area of the rats' brains was suppressing or erasing the memory of the fear response. To determine which of these possibilities was the correct one, LeDoux carried out a delicate surgical operation on the rats, damaging a tiny part of their forebrains. The result? The rats not only did not lose their fear of the sound; they actually remained afraid much longer than the control group of rats that had not been operated upon. It thus appears that the frontal region of the rat brain helps suppress and control the emotional memories generated by the amygdala. This neurofeedback process actually makes a lot of sense. An emotional response may be useful at first—often even necessary for physical survival—but will eventually lose its usefulness. If rats reacted in fear and terror every single time they perceived the same stimulus, they might in some circumstances starve to death or be unable to reach a mate in order to breed. Emotional responses to certain situations can have great survival value, but so can the ability to override or suppress those responses.

This doesn't just apply to rats. Millions of Americans suffer from phobias of various kinds, from recurring panic attacks, and from PTSD. Nearly a million people, 85 percent of them women, suffer from agoraphobia, the fear of being in public places. Panic disorders are fairly common, affecting 1–2 percent of the population, and tend to run in families. What these conditions all have in common is an uncontrollable fear response to otherwise benign situations. "You can tell phobics all day long, 'This will not hurt you,'" LeDoux has said, "but they don't believe it."

It's a frustrating experience for the person afflicted with a phobia or panic attacks, as I myself know. When I have a panic attack, I know perfectly well how absurd my reaction is. I may even find myself talking aloud to myself: "C'mon, this is ridiculous. All I'm doing is driving over this bridge. I've driven over it hundreds of times before. Nothing is going to happen. I know it. So stop this right now!" I grit my teeth, focus fiercely on the road right in front of my car, stay hyperaware of any cars nearby, and just drive across the bridge. Minutes later I am perfectly calm, composed, even feeling happy.

What's happened? Something, it seems, has gone awry with the intricate circuitry that allows an area in my forebrain to modulate the fear reaction my amygdala is pumping out. In my particular case, I frankly have no idea what the actual physiological or neurological breakdown may be. Certain stressful situations still seem to trigger my panic attacks. As I noted earlier, I can no longer get up in front of an audience to teach a writing class, give a lecture, or do a book reading without experiencing at least a mild form of anxiety attack. It's never stopped me from teaching, lecturing, or publicizing my newest book; the unreasoning fear usually dissipates within a few minutes. But why the occasional panic attacks when I drive over a bridge? I almost never experience driving a car as stressful, and ninety-nine times out of a hundred that also goes for driving across bridges. Why did I have a truly terrifying panic attack while walking across the Golden Gate Bridge with my wife and her best friend? I don't know, but Joseph LeDoux may be providing us all with clues.

THE BEGINNINGS OF EMOTIONS

Humans, like other animals, express emotions from the day they are born. Pain, hunger, fear, and satisfaction are all accompanied by vocal cries or facial expressions that most parents quickly learn to recognize. However, these early emotional expressions are not connected to any cognitive functions. A human infant is simply not old enough to think; the brain has not developed enough for that to happen.

By the time a child is twelve to eighteen months old, he or she has begun to speak. Language, as we'll see in the next chapter, presupposes an ability to connect a symbol—a word or phrase like "Mama," "Dada," "cat"—with a nonverbal concept. That means thought. During the same period, the child is also forging the brain connections between thought and emotion. Researchers usually follow the development of these connections by studying the infant's facial expressions. The facial expressions, says psychologist Nathan Fox, mirror the development of a central emotional system in the brain. Fox, at the University of Maryland in College Park, has studied the brains of human infants as they express emotions. He believes that in humans the amygdala evaluates sensory information and makes the decision to either approach or withdraw from the person, event, or object that is the source of a sensory stimulus. The infant's brain furiously develops its vast network of synaptic connections, and the amygdala forges neural links to the frontal lobes, where high-order cognitive processing will take place. As this occurs, the amygdala begins forming what Fox calls the "primary" emotions of anger, fear, disgust, interest, joy, and sadness and their associated emotional memories.

Fox has also found changes in the electrical activity of infants' brains as this process occurs. During the 1980s, he and his colleagues used an EEG (electroencephalogram)-like imaging device to record the electrical activity of the brains of infants. They found that the electrical activity in the brain's left cerebral hemisphere increased when the child experienced "positive" emotions, such as joy, interest, and satisfaction. The electrical activity in the brain's right hemisphere increased when the child experienced "negative" emotions, such as fear, anger, and sadness. The most striking increases in right-hemisphere activity, says Fox, take place when an infant is crying. The largest surges in left-hemisphere electrical activity occur when the child is smiling.

THE WOMAN WHO KNOWS NOT FEAR

Antonio Damasio and his wife, Hanna, work at the University of Iowa College of Medicine in Iowa City. For years they have used a combination of advanced imaging technologies and old-fashioned psychological and neurological testing to ferret out fascinating insights into the way the brain works. Their efforts have helped increase our understanding of the connections between the brain and language, memory, and emotions. The Damasios usually work with people who have suffered strokes, brain injuries, or other traumas that have damaged or destroyed specific areas of their brains. As a result, these people have lost certain mental faculties that we all usually take for granted. Hanna Damasio creates positron-emission tomography (PET) or magnetic resonance imaging (MRI) images that precisely pinpoint the damaged regions. She and her husband and their colleagues then give the patients a series of tests; the tests reveal the nature and extent of the consequences of the brain damage.

One of the patients that the Damasios have worked with is a woman, S.M. Born in 1964, she has been described by Antonio Damasio as "nice, cooperative, and intelligent." S.M. suffered from a rare disease that had left calcium deposits in her brain's amygdala. We all have two amygdalas, one in each temporal lobe. S.M.'s disease had destroyed both of hers.

Several people studied by the Damasios and their colleagues Daniel Tranel and Rolf Adolphs are no longer able to recognize formerly familiar faces. It may be a husband of thirty years, but his face is now as unfamiliar as that of a stranger. Indeed, a patient with this peculiar form of memory loss, called face agnosia, cannot even recognize his or her own face in a mirror. The person may know intellectually that it must be his or her face in the mirror, but there is no feeling of familiarity with it. These people have suffered damage to the left visual association cortex, a part of the brain that processes visual data coming from the primary visual cortex. Despite this loss of intellectual comprehension, all these patients were still able to "read" facial expressions of emotion. Scowls, grins, expressions of surprise—all were instantly identifiable.

As we saw earlier, Joseph LeDoux has provided powerful evidence of the role of the amygdala in the formation of fear memories. Researchers also know that the amygdala in animals plays a role in social behavior. For example, when you reach down and gently rub the side of your pet cat, the neurons in the animal's amygdala become active. The same response occurs when one cat rubs another cat's side. In humans, though, the role of the amygdala has remained somewhat uncertain.

The Damasios and their colleagues have been studying S.M. because of her remarkable inability to experience fear. To start with, they found that she cannot "read" facial expressions of emotion. In one experiment, the researchers showed S.M. a series of photographs of faces. Each photo showed a human face expressing an emotion, including anger, fear, disgust, happiness, sadness, and surprise. Several pictures also showed faces with neutral expressions; these were "control" pictures. The researchers asked S.M. to pick an adjective that described the emotion on each face.

The woman had no problem describing most of the emotional expressions. Only one stumped her: fear. She verbally stumbled about, looking for the right word to describe the expression she was looking at. But she could not.

Even more fascinating was her response to another experiment. S.M. was asked to look at her face in a mirror and, while doing so, form an expression of fear. Once again, she was stumped. She would raise her eyebrows, wriggle them about, twist her mouth into different shapes. It was all for naught. She finally stopped her grimacing and said, "I can't do it." The reason, of course, was that she did not have a memory of what the fear experience feels like. She cannot feel the emotion we call fear. And because she has no comprehension of what that emotion feels like, she cannot make the facial expression that reflects it.

The Damasios also carried out another experiment with S.M. and a group of other people, some of them patients with brain damage. They were shown photos of faces. Each face presented a mixture of emotional expressions, as most faces do most of the time. The subjects were to rate how much of any given emotion was present on each face using a scale running from 1 to 5. All of the other people in the subject group easily "read" the emotions in each photograph. Their ratings were all quite similar. But S.M. could recognize only one emotion at a time in each face. She could not detect the natural complexity of human emotional expressions. The one other exception was fear. Once again, she could not detect fear at all in any of the facial expressions.

S.M.'s peculiar problem sheds new light on the mystery of emotions. If this woman had a gun put to her head, Antonio Damasio has said, she would know intellectually that she should be afraid. But she would not *feel fear*. At the same time, she can both experience other emotions and recognize their expression in other people's faces. But she can recognize only one facial expression of emotion at a time per face. According to Damasio, S.M.'s deficiency reveals that the brain has separate subsystems for identifying faces and for identifying facial *expressions*. The brain normally brings these two pieces of perception together in a seamless and unconscious fashion. We are not aware that it's happening; we just know our father by his face, and we know that he's pissed as hell. Researchers, thanks to S.M., now know that the amygdala plays a major role in making this happen. Should it be damaged or destroyed, the links between facial identity and awareness of fear are erased.

THOUGHT AND EMOTIONS

The philosophical position known as dualism holds that the brain and the mind are two different entities. The current version of dualism springs from the writings of the French philosopher René Descartes. Descartes believed, among other things, that the brain was the seat of reason, language, morality, and the spirit. The body, on the other hand, was the location of such "lower" functions as instincts and emotions. We'll look at dualism in somewhat more depth later on. However, suffice to say at this point that dualism has had far-reaching consequences for the cognitive sciences. Like any long-accepted paradigm for reality, it has silently and subtly shaped the way researchers have studied the brain.

The dualism paradigm created a set of unspoken assumptions, and those assumptions precluded certain questions. In fact, it led most brain researchers to simply ignore entire areas of research. Imagine, for example, if astronomers had never bothered to use telescopes to examine the planets because "everyone knew" that the planets were just moving dots of light in the sky. That is actually what the state of astronomical affairs was like until the first decade of the seventeenth century. The kinds of lenses needed to make telescopes had been known about for decades, if not longer. Early crude telescopes had also been around for many years. It took the first tentative shifts in the European worldview, nudged forward by Copernicus's writings, to make the difference. Galileo Galilei had been captivated by Copernicus's book *De Revolutionibus Orbium Celestium* and its implications for the nature of reality. He seized upon the telescope as an instrument that would prove the truth of Copernicus's assertions. It did.

The new medical imaging technologies are making the same kinds of changes possible in the study of the brain and emotions. Philosophers and, more recently, psychologists examined emotions and their effect on behavior, but they did so by observing what people say and do. Descriptive methods of study can only go so far, and few moved past external observation and description into neurological exploration and experimentation. As far as human emotions and behavior were concerned, the brain remained an unopened black box.

For example, most scientists accepted the long-established philosophical premise that emotions and rational thought were two entirely separate activities. This was a dualistic assumption, of course, and under the circumstances quite understandable. To carry out biological studies of human emotions was something long presumed to be much too difficult to ever pull off. But the new brain-imaging machines have now given researchers the means to shine a light on the inner workings of the human brain. They are now able to ferret out the brain's emotional circuitry and reveal the intimate connections—the physical connections—between our emotions and our thoughts.

Emotions are neither mystical nor ephemeral. As we've seen, they are the brain's way of interpreting our "gut" reactions to the world beyond our skin. The connection between our emotions and our thoughts is quite real and very important. For example, brain researchers can now confirm what many psychologists and psychotherapists have long suspected and even assumed: Emotional memories are permanent. They become ingrained in the brain's circuitry. We may be able to suppress emotional memories, sometimes for years; but they are always there, stored away and waiting for the right trigger to launch them into our consciousness once again.

Another example: Cognitive scientists now have evidence that emotions are an essential part of our ability to reason. Contrary to the position of many philosophers and poets through the centuries, we cannot reason effectively without the input from emotions. In a similar vein, the kinds of emotions we sometimes call "gut feelings" or "intuition" are essential for making rational decisions. This, too, sounds contradictory. But the neurological evidence is unmistakable.

THE NEW NEUROBIOLOGY OF EMOTIONS

In his acclaimed 1994 book *Descartes' Error*, Antonio Damasio sketches out a new neurobiology of emotions. This new understanding of the brain's emotional circuitry has come about in large part through the use of the new brain-imaging technologies.

Three groups of patients studied by Damasio have led him to formulate this new map of the brain's emotional networks. The first group are people called neglect patients. They have suffered damage to the right somatosensory cortex that has left the left side of their bodies paralyzed. Despite this paralysis, neglect patients have no awareness that anything is wrong. If you ask one if she can move her left arm, she will reply, "Of course I can." If you then ask her to do so, she will say, "Gladly," and nothing happens. If you say, "Well? Why didn't you move your left arm?" she will come up with some kind of excuse. "I didn't feel like it, after all." "Give me some time; I'll get around to it." "That's not my arm. That's my husband's arm! How can you expect me to move my husband's arm?"

The phenomenon of the neglect patient occurs only when a specific part of the right somatosensory cortex is damaged. The particular region involved is responsible for processing information from several different external senses, including pain, temperature, and touch, as well as the senses that detect the position of the limbs, head, and trunk. This particular part of the somatosensory cortex, along with other regions, creates an integrated map of the body's current state of being— where it is, what it's feeling, and where it's headed in space. If the corresponding physical location in the left somatosensory cortex is damaged, neglect does not occur, for the right hemisphere is dominant in this case. Neglect patients, in other words, have lost their brains' internal maps of their own bodies. The brain of a particular patient just mentioned, for example, cannot and does not know where her left arm is in space or in relation to the rest of her body. So she invents excuses for not moving her arm.

A second group of patients has also given Damasio clues to the workings of emotions in the brain. These people have suffered damage to a small region in the brain's prefrontal cortexes. These regions of the frontal lobes lie above the eyes and right behind the forehead. All these patients have had significant changes in their personalities after the damage. One such patient Damasio identifies as "Eliot." Eliot now lives a life in emotional neutral. He never expresses any sadness or impatience about life's difficulties or his situation. Eliot also has serious difficulty making what we would call ethical decisions. Most of us, faced with a choice of buying the chocolate bar or slipping it into our jacket pocket and walking out of the store, have no trouble understanding which is the ethically wrong decision. However, if we were to then suffer the kind of brain damage that Eliot has, we would suddenly have a great deal of difficulty figuring it out. Damasio believes that Eliot, and others like him, reveal a connection between emotions and feelings and the ability to make rational and ethical decisions.

The third group of patients are like S.M. Their amygdalas are destroyed. They cannot recognize fear either in themselves or others. This deficit, like running in emotional neutral for the people in the second group, has a profound impact on a person's ability to make reasonable decisions.

But wait. Isn't decision making a "rational faculty?" One of the "higher" faculties praised by Descartes? How can there possibly be a connection between decision making and a "lower" impulse like emotions?

Well, says Damasio and many other brain researchers, Descartes was wrong. Thought and emotion are inextricably bound together. In fact, the ability to make decisions that are rational and ethical is not possible without the ability to experience emotions. According to Damasio and his colleagues, the brain's wiring diagram for emotions works something like this:

1. First comes a perception of some kind. Let's suppose it's the sight of an angry, hostile stranger at your front door. The neural signals created by this visual perception first travel to the thalamus, the early processing station for sensory information.

2. From the thalamus the signals travel to the visual cortex for primary processing.

3. From there the processed information goes in two different directions, to the prefrontal cortexes at the front of the frontal lobes and to structures in the limbic system, such as the amygdala. Information processed in the prefrontal cortex also flows downward along another neural pathway into the limbic system. The amygdala and the prefrontal cortexes evaluate and process this information conceptually. In particular, the amygdala turns out to be Emotion Central, providing the first quick and dirty evaluations of the sensory inputs' potential emotional significance. They essentially compare it with data from earlier experiences and create a neural response. In this case, you do not recognize the face; it is a stranger; you do recognize the facial expressions of anger and potential violence.

4. The response information from the amygdala now races down two different neural pathways. One leads to the brain stem. The other pathway leads to the hypothalamus. The brain stem commands the release of various neurotransmitter chemicals in the brain. These chemicals change the way some neural networks in the brain work and activate others. The hypothalamus helps control the autonomic nervous system and the body's endocrine system. The endocrine system is the collection of glands that secrete hormones and includes the adrenals, thyroid, parathyroid gland, pituitary gland, pineal gland, and the ovaries. The release of appropriate hormones puts the body into a state of alert—your stomach and intestinal muscles tighten up; your skin becomes cold, clammy, almost prickly; the muscles in your back, arms, and legs tense up; your heart starts beating fast.

5. The body itself now returns signals to the brain, reporting its altered state. This information travels to the right somatosensory cortex for evaluation and response. Meanwhile, the neurotransmitters released by signals sent to the brain stem have already started to alter the status of numerous neural networks and subsystems. This chain of activities, in turn, alters how your brain handles the data that have arrived at the somatosensory cortex. If this were an old friend at the door, your bodily reaction and subsequent responses by your brain would be very different from the ones you are having now.

An emotion, says Damasio, is thus produced by the combination of two sets of signals. One comes back to the brain from the body, reporting on the body's state of being. The other is generated in the brain itself by the conceptual evaluations of the stimulus by the prefrontal cortex and amygdala. The collection of alterations in the state of the mind and body which these neural circuits detect is the essence of an emotion. The feeling that results—fear, in this case—is our experience of these changes.

We learn and remember a set of movements to ride a bicycle or the patterns of light, shade, texture, and color that equal our father's face. In the same way, our brains learn and remember these collections of changes in the state of the body and mind. The emotions that psychologists call primary—fear, hunger, anger, sadness, satisfaction, anticipation—become deeply ingrained early in life in the brain's emotional circuitry. Other emotions, such as shyness or silliness, are variations on the primary emotions that we learn later.

THE SHORTCUT

This five-step route for neural information that creates what we call emotions is not the only one, however. In 1991, LeDoux and his associates at New York University uncovered another pathway—a shortcut. Primitive emotions like fear, LeDoux discovered, can often travel a direct route from the thalamus down to the amygdala. This pathway completely bypasses any preliminary processing in the cerebral cortex.

I once worked in a bookstore in Southern California. My manager, a young man in his late twenties named Ted, was a Vietnam veteran. One Monday morning, Ted arrived at the bookstore with a story about himself. He chuckled as he related it, but I later realized that it was one of those "it wasn't funny at the time" kinds of laughs. He and his wife had gone down to Los Angeles that weekend to visit friends. As they and their friends had been walking along the sidewalk talking, a car going by had suddenly backfired with a loud *pop-pop-pop!* Said Ted, "It was the strangest thing—but all of a sudden I found myself *coming up* from a rolling crouch on the sidewalk!" More than twenty-five years later, I still remember the bemused expression on his face as he told the story. "That happens sometimes," he added. "A sound like gunfire, and *wham!*—I react without thinking."

LeDoux can explain that reaction. A neural pathway running from the thalamus carries that kind of information to the amygdala two to three times faster than the route that first goes to the cortex and then back down into the brain. This high-speed route, LeDoux believes, makes it possible for the amygdala to make an almost instantaneous judgment as to whether that sound is something to fear or to be ignored. And it happens literally before we have time to think about it. Cognition and emotion do interact—the work by the Damasios is proof of that—but sometimes cognition lags behind the primary emotional processing.

In the case of my old bookstore manager, this shortcut to the amygdala processed some aural information before he knew intellectually what the sound was. Also, it wrongly identified the sound. He reacted as if it were gunshots. Those are good reactions in a jungle, surrounded by people shooting at you. Ted had learned that lesson well. Perhaps too well. His exaggerated response to the backfiring car may well have been a symptom of PTSD.

PTSD AND THE AMYGDALA

PTSD, panic disorder, obsessions, compulsions, and phobias are the external manifestations of brain responses gone awry. In the last several years, a number of researchers have been using PET and MRI to make images of these neural perturbations in the brain. Scott Rauch is one such researcher. Rauch is a psychiatrist at Harvard University Medical School and Massachusetts General Hospital. He and his associates have worked with people suffering from PTSD and studied their brains during their episodes using PET scans.

For one study, Rauch first had the subjects write some narratives that invoked a neutral-feeling scene for them—perhaps a short description of canoeing on a calm lake on a quiet morning or washing the dishes. Meanwhile, the researcher and his colleagues enlisted other volunteers to write vivid, disturbing narratives that would trigger the PTSD feelings in the subjects.

As in other PET scan tests to pinpoint functional areas of the brain, Rauch and his colleagues first carried out a "baseline" test. For this experiment, each volunteer lay in the PET imager while his or her neutral narrative was read. As this happened, each would inhale air laced with radioactively tagged carbon dioxide to provide the positrons for the PET image. Then each person waited twenty minutes while the radioisotope decayed into indetectability. Then each would listen to the "trigger" narrative, the disturbing story or account that would set off their PTSD symptoms.

Rauch and his colleagues discovered that several different areas of the brain became active during the PTSD attacks. They included the posterior orbitofrontal cortex, the part of the frontal lobes lying right behind the forehead; the anterior cingulate cortex, which is above and behind the orbitofrontal area; the anterior temporal cortex, part of the temporal lobes right in front of the ears; and the insular cortex, which lies in a fold of neural tissue deep inside the cerebral cortex. These four areas are also known to be important processing areas for the emotion we call anxiety and are often called the "worry circuit." Rauch's PET images show that most of these regions are very active during OCD attacks, panic attacks, and phobias, all of which are types of anxiety disorders.

In the case of PTSD, however, the PET scans revealed that it was primarily the right-hemisphere regions of the "worry circuit" that lit up. This appears to confirm Nathan Fox's findings in infants, that the right cerebral hemisphere is more active than the left during distressing emotions.

Another very active brain structure during PTSD symptoms was, yes, the amygdala. Rauch thinks this makes sense. PTSD, he has been quoted as saying, is "the vivid evocation of a painful, haunting memory." Moreover, many PTSD victims insist that these memories are more than just memories. They are so vivid, so powerful, that the sufferers feel as if they are reliving the events all over again. Many PTSD sufferers experience these memories visually. They suffer visual "flashbacks" that are more than hallucinatory; they *feel real*. It turns out that Rauch's PET scans reveal high levels of activity in the visual cortexes of people suffering from PTSD symptoms.

Another PET revelation was a sharp depression of activity in the brain's language regions. Rauch says this dovetails with another common aspect of PTSD. "Patients have difficulty putting words to these emotions," he has said, "and so have trouble dealing with the experiences."

IMAGES OF OBSESSION

Rauch and his colleagues have also conducted PET and MRI studies of people suffering from OCD. One study by Rauch and his colleagues involved exposing eight men and women to the very objects that triggered their OCD reactions. The researchers carefully worked everything out beforehand with the subjects. They not only had the volunteers' full approval but also cooperation. One woman, for example, explained that a dirty towel would trigger her obsessions about contamination and germs and provoke a compulsive need to wash her hands again and again. That became her trigger stimulus, while a freshly laundered towel was her neutral stimulus (an object that would not trigger her obsession). A man in the study had obsessions that centered on a fear of becoming violent and hurting someone. He and the researchers settled on a photo of his dog as a neutral stimulus. A photograph of a serial killer was the trigger stimulus.

For the baseline part of the experiment, the subjects would lie inside the PET imager as they held or looked at the neutral trigger object. The woman with the soiled washcloth obsession, for example, held the clean cloth as a PET image was made. Then the researchers gave her the dirty washcloth. As soon as she told them her obsession had really kicked in, the researchers took a second series of PET images. Holding a towel while both images were made was essential to the success of this test. It made it possible for the researchers to identify the parts of the brain activated by just holding a towel and those parts that lit up because the woman was obsessing about a dirty towel.

Rauch and his colleagues discovered that, as with PTSD sufferers, the "worry circuit" lit up in the brains of the people with OCD. In their case, there was no hemispheric asymmetry to the activity. The worry-circuit regions in both hemispheres were active. Another part of the brain that becomes active during OCD and panic attacks is the locus ceruleus. This is a small nucleus of neurons in the brain stem that secretes the neurotransmitter noradrenaline. In the body, noradrenaline also functions as a hormone. In both the body and brain, noradrenaline is released when a person is under stress.

Rauch also discovered that the visual cortex and those parts of the brain involved with language also became active during OCD attacks and panic reactions. He thinks this is connected to how the subjects experience their obsessions. Some people, he has said, "see with their mind's eye or hear with their mind's ear" as they undergo their obsessive and compulsive feelings. For example, a woman who feels the obsessive need to wash her hands may be subconsciously saying to herself, "Wash your hands, wash your hands, wash your hands, wash your hands, wash your hands . . ." That kind of brain activity will cause her language centers to light up in a PET scan.

Rauch also has carried out similar studies with people who suffer from simple phobias, particularly excessive fear of snakes and tarantulas. In these experiments, the PET scans revealed increased activity in the tactile cortex. This is the part of the motor and somatosensory cortexes that processes the sense of touch. When the subjects described their phobias, Rauch says, they mostly talked about their fear of touching or being touched by the animals. So it's not surprising that the areas of the brain that process touch sensations were active even though the animals never came close to the subjects.

AN IMAGE OF PANIC

Rauch is not the only researcher using the new brain-imaging technologies to study emotions in the brain. At the University of Washington School of Medicine in Seattle, Stephen Dager and his colleagues have been working with people who suffer from panic attacks. Dager has focused on one particular symptom of panic attacks: hyperventilation. Hyperventilation is abnormally fast or deep breathing that results in the loss of carbon dioxide from the blood. It causes a drop in blood pressure, tingling of the extremities, and sometimes fainting.

For this experiment the researchers worked with two groups of people. One group were patients being treated for panic attacks. The other group were people who did not suffer from panic attacks. Dager and his associates had both groups make themselves hyperventilate by breathing rapidly and deeply. As they did so, the members of both groups had images made of their brains using a technique called functional proton spectroscopic imaging.

Dager discovered a brain difference between the people suffering from panic attacks and those who didn't. Specifically, the insular cortex in those with panic disorder was much more active than in those without the disorder. Dager and his colleagues are now looking to see if other areas in the brain are also excessively active in people with panic disorder.

THE CHEMICAL CONNECTION

While Dager and his associates at the University of Washington track down the regions in the brain that play a role in panic attacks, a research team in Toronto, Canada, is pinpointing the brain chemical that is the

likely trigger. It's another link in the chain of discoveries that may eventually tell me—and millions of other people—why we sometimes have
these episodes of overwhelming fear.

Jacques Bradwejn is a psychiatrist at Toronto's Clarke Institute of
Psychiatry. In 1987 he and a team of researchers discovered that a brain
chemical called cholecystokinin (or CCK) is one of the main biological
sources of the panic reaction. CCK is a neurotransmitter, one of the
many chemicals in the brain that carries signals across synapses from
one neuron to another. Different neurons release different neurotransmitters to send the signals across the synaptic gap. Some use dopamine
as their neurotransmitter; others, serotonin or one of the endorphins.
Researchers have already discovered and classified literally dozens of
different neurotransmitters in the brain and nervous system. They are
not distributed randomly, but are used by neurons found in distinct
brain sites.

CCK is used as a neurotransmitter by clusters of neurons in the limbic system. It's part of a complex feedback loop that normally regulates
memory storage and retrieval as well as arousal. According to Bradwejn,
when this delicate system of neuronal messages carried by CCK is
somehow disrupted, the result is frequent panic attacks.

Panic attacks of the kind that I experienced daily for several months
in 1989 usually last about twenty minutes. A typical sufferer will experience them an average of eight times a week—about one a day. And one
a day is plenty. It isn't long before the person begins to wonder not if the
next one will hit but when. Will it happen as I drive to work? As I walk
down the aisles in the grocery store? As I sit in church? On the bus? In
class? When friends are visiting? When I'm visiting friends? Many people who suffer from chronic panic attacks start looking for excuses to
stay home, to not go outside or see people. The disorder thus grows into
agoraphobia, the fear of being in any public place. You just don't know
when the attack will happen again.

The experience itself, as I related at the beginning of this chapter, is
utterly terrifying. Some people think they're having a heart attack; they
truly believe they are about to die. Your heart pounds furiously, your
skin becomes clammy, you feel almost uncontrollably dizzy, your hands
sweat, you feel as if you may suffocate at any moment.

Though CCK is now known to be a major source of panic disorder,
researchers still don't know how it does what it does. There may be a
genetic component, however, since the receptor, or chemical "keyhole,"

on neurons which CCK plugs into must be created by a particular gene. Researchers have recently isolated a gene that codes for the production of CCK itself. It is also known that people with panic disorder are extremely sensitive to CCK. During panic attacks, the CCK receptors on the neurons that respond to the neurotransmitter are "ingesting" more than the brain can deal with.

The question is, however, is this a matter of too much CCK or not enough? Or too many CCK receptors or not enough? Any of these could be the cause. For example, the neurons in the CCK system could be releasing too much of the chemical, overwhelming the CCK receptors. Alternatively, there could be a problem with the gene or genes that code for the receptors. Perhaps the neurons have fewer CCK receptors than normal; they would be overwhelmed not by an overproduction of CCK but by the normal amount. Then again, the neurons that produce CCK may not make enough of it most of the time. The receptors that are present become more and more sensitive to compensate. When the neurons suddenly produce a lot of CCK during a stressful or emotional situation, the oversensitive receptors get knocked out of whack. The result: a panic attack, PTSD symptoms, or a resurgence of a phobic reaction.

Further complicating matters is that there are actually two kinds of CCK receptors on neurons. One type, called CCK-A, usually acts to calm people down. The second type, CCK-B, acts to promote feelings of anxiety that can lead to panic attacks. So, do I have too many CCK-B receptors or not enough CCK-A receptors?

ACCEPTANCE, ANGER, anticipation, disgust, fear, grief, happiness, joy, sadness, surprise—we live our lives immersed in a sea of emotions. Sometimes we don't consciously feel them; usually we do. They are always there, however. We would not be human without them. For one thing, what would we have to talk about, write about, sing about, or dream about if there were no emotions?

And another thing: If Antonio Damasio and his colleagues are right, we would not even be able to think without them.

CHAPTER 10

THE MYSTERY OF LANGUAGE

MY MOTHER was eleven years old when she came to the United States in 1937. Her father, Desai Farkas, had come from Budapest to New York City a year earlier. He got a job as a tool and die maker, found an apartment in Queens, saved his money, and then sent for his wife and two daughters.

My mother had spoken Hungarian, her native tongue, her entire life. She knew no other languages. Suddenly she found herself uprooted from her home and living in a new city surrounded by strange new people speaking a totally unfamiliar language. She was entering the equivalent of junior high school. She didn't speak a word of English.

Today she shrugs. "I learned," she says. "I learned pretty fast. I didn't have much choice, since everyone else but me spoke English." Nearly sixty years later, her English is flawless. She speaks like a native, though strangers who meet her for the first time can still hear a trace of that Hungarian accent.

My maternal grandmother, on the other hand, always spoke English with a thick accent. Her grandchildren found it charming; even today, years after her death, my siblings and I will sometimes imitate that trilling accent with which she spoke and feel a great fondness for her.

Why the difference in accents, though, between my mother and her mother? Why did Antonia Farkas learn English so well, while Augusta Farkas did not?

Linguists have long known that the older a person is when she learns a new language, the harder it is to pick up and retain. Numerous studies reveal that the cutoff is around age ten or so. After that point, learning new languages—while not impossible—becomes progressively harder. My mother and her sister were still young enough to learn a second language with relative ease. My grandmother and grandfather were not. Today brain researchers know the why of this cutoff date. And a whole lot more.

The brain is the playing field of language. The new imaging technologies have proved particularly useful in studying the connections between the two. Researchers are also using more traditional methods to explore the brain's language connections. These time-tested methods include lesion studies and microelectrode readings. This work has not only confirmed the linguistic role of several cerebral regions long known to neurologists but has also uncovered new brain regions involved with language.

THE LINGUISTIC BRAIN

Brain scientists since the mid–eighteenth century have known that several different parts of the brain are involved with language. Three of them are the somatosensory cortex, the motor cortex, and the primary visual cortex. The somatosensory cortex has deep neural connections to the brain's speech and hearing regions. The motor cortex also plays an important role in language, since it controls the movements of the lips, jaw, tongue, and pharynx—essential to vocal language—and the arms, hands, fingers—vital for signed languages. The processing regions in the primary visual cortex at the back of the occipital lobe also play a role in language, whether verbal, signed, or written. The visual cortex processes the written symbols that constitute writing and the hand signals used in signed languages and passes that information on to other parts of the brain. And because we receive the vast majority of our information about the world through our sense of sight, the visual processing area provides the brain's higher-level association and decision-making regions with a vast amount of information that contributes to language.

The other previously known language areas are located, for most people, in the brain's left hemisphere—the dominant cerebral hemisphere for language in 99 percent of right-handed people and well over 60 percent of left-handers. The great majority of left-handed people who do not have a language-dominant left hemisphere have their language centers equally distributed in both hemispheres. Only a small percentage of people have dominant right-brain hemispheres for language, and most of them suffered some kind of brain damage in infancy. The brain in infants and young children is still growing and developing, so it quickly adapts to such situations. Other structures in the nondamaged hemisphere are thus able to assume language functions.

The language regions known to exist (for most people) in the left hemisphere are Broca's area, Heschl's gyrus, and Wernicke's area. Broca's area lies in the lower back part of the left frontal lobe, along the inner part of the left frontal ridge, the third ridge of brain tissue on the left frontal lobe. It was discovered by Paul Broca in 1861. Most brain scientists and linguists have long believed that Broca's area is the brain's center for encoding speech.

Heschl's gyri are ridges or folds of brain tissues lying along the upper part of the brain's left temporal lobe. Named for the nineteenth-century Austrian pathologist Richard L. Heschl, this is a major region for auditory perception and therefore plays an important role in verbal (as opposed to signed) language.

Wernicke's area was discovered by Karl Wernicke in 1874. Wernicke worked with people suffering from various forms of aphasia, a difficulty in speaking caused by brain damage. Some of Wernicke's patients had problems with their syntax. That is, they could not speak grammatically or understand what other people said. When these patients later died, Wernicke did autopsies of their brain. He discovered that the left temporal and parietal lobes of these people had scar tissue and other damage. The area of the brain that he identified with this aphasia has come to be known as Wernicke's area. It lies along the upper regions of the left temporal and parietal lobes, behind Broca's area. A brain region lying just below Wernicke's area is involved in the control of the hand movements of sign language.

Wernicke's and Broca's discoveries gave scientists the first glimpses of the distributed nature of language function in the brain. The brain seemed to have no single location where language is created or stored. Instead, it looked as if different parts of the brain control different aspects of speech and language. Broca's area, for example, seemed to be the region that controlled speech production. Wernicke's area, on the other hand, dealt with language comprehension and grammar.

It turns out to be not quite that simple, of course.

But what *is* remarkably simple is the way we all come to language. For no matter who we are, where we are born, what culture we are born into, or what our mother tongue may be, we all create language pretty much the same way and at the same time. All humans have brains that are wired for language, and the wiring is the same for everyone.

WIRED FOR WORDS

Infants do not begin their journey into the world of language with random steps. Decades of scientific observation and experimentation have revealed that they create language in an orderly fashion. They follow a specific sequence of events that starts with biological noises and ends with first words. Moreover, this sequence is universal; human infants follow the timetable no matter what their mother tongue may be. While different researchers offer different variations, the general timetable for infant language acquisition appears in table 10.1. It goes like this:

- During the first several weeks, the infant cries. Crying is at first undifferentiated. Then the infant's cries become specific—hunger, fear, sleepy, dirty diaper, and so on. At this point the sounds are all still biological in nature. They have no true linguistic nature.
- By the time the infant is about one to two months old, she begins making sounds that sound a little like vowels. At first these are formed at the front of her vocal tract; these are the kinds of sounds you make by pursing your lips: *ooo*. By the time she is two to three months old, she begins cooing.
- When the baby is about four months old, she begins making vowel-like sounds farther back in the mouth, like *aaah*. She also starts to laugh, chuckle, and gurgle. By six months, she is able to imitate the sounds made by her parents and change pitch and inflection.
- From six to eight months of age, the baby begins to babble. Babbling is the repetition of simple vowel-consonant combinations such as *mamamama, babababa,* and *dada.* By now the child is imitating the words spoken by the parents and may well understand what some words mean. She is already beginning to connect verbal symbols with nonverbal concepts. So, for example, the infant now understands that the word "Mama" means her mother.
- Sometime between a year and eighteen months, the child begins speaking her own first words. It is at this point that the child has clearly begun to master true language.

Month:	Language Stage
0–1	Crying stage
1–2	Crying and cooing
2–3	↓
3–4	↓
4–5	Laughing and gurgling
5–6	↓
6–7	Repeating sounds/babbling
7–8	↓
8–9	↓
9–10	Repeating words/first words
10–11	↓
11–12	↓
12–13	True speech begins
13–14	↓
14–15	↓
15–16	↓
16–17	↓
17–18	↓

TABLE 10.1.   A Timetable for Language

By eighteen months, the average normally developing child has a vocabulary of about 20–50 words and can understand as many as 250. By the age of two a child has a working vocabulary of 200 words; by age three, a thousand. Not only is the child's brain undergoing a continuing tremendous growth in synaptic connections; a "bootstrap" effect is also taking place. The more words a child learns and the more sophisticated the child's grammatical ability becomes, the more words the child is *able* to learn and comprehend. Once it begins, language ability feeds itself.

But *how* does it begin? More to the point, how can any child begin from no language knowledge at all and within eighteen months be speaking intelligently? The answer, again, lies in the brain.

Over and over again, we have seen a consistent pattern to the brain's operations. That pattern is—pattern. From visual perception to detecting music, from body movements to remembering faces, from learning to ride a bicycle to learning words, the brain looks for *patterns*. The brain is, first and foremost, a pattern detector. The patterns may be visual or aural, body movements or shapes, disruptions in space or in temporal sequence. If it's a pattern, a rhythm, the brain will notice it and do something with it.

Human infants can smell the difference between Mom and some other human. They can identify their mothers' faces soon after birth and distinguish between the different faces of different people. Infants can tell the difference between sweet and bitter tastes. They prefer sweet (sweet equals sugar; sugar is high-energy food) and hate bitter. (Bitter often means poisonous; avoid it.)

Infants can clearly distinguish different sounds. Moreover, some sounds are more important than others. Babies are attuned to high-pitched sounds, for example. They prefer them to those of a lower pitch and respond to them quickly. It is no surprise that when parents and other adults talk to infants, their "baby talk" is almost always in a high pitch. Human infants are also particularly sensitive to speech sounds. They will respond much more quickly to sounds like *baba* or *dada* or *paba* than to random, nonlinguistic sounds.

The noises an infant makes during the first few weeks of its life are *reflexive noises*. But even these cries of hunger, fear, or pain are rhythmic—a natural consequence of the way sounds are made in the vocal tract as the vocal chords rhythmically open and close during various kinds of cries. This also varies the pitch. Rhythm, pitch patterns, and modulation of the exhaled breath by the vocal fold are all basic characteristics of verbal speech. So not only are our brains predisposed to detect patterns and rhythms in nature; our very vocal apparatus naturally produces rhythmic, patterned sounds even before we begin speaking. Next come whispers, growls, squeals, yells, and howls. Infants also begin making sounds that resemble vowels.

By the time infants are six to eight months old, the muscles of their mouths, tongues, and lips are mature enough to create sounds that resemble speech sounds. Their brains are learning by observing, remembering—and repeating. So they repeat what they hear. The babies begin babbling, stringing language sounds together in clear patterns. The patterns don't yet have meaning, but that is soon to come. Babbling has the rhythmic texture of true language. Infants are now not only making the right sounds but also making them with the correct rhythms. What's more, infants at this point are using *selected* speech sounds. When they are only a few weeks old, all infants make all possible language sounds, from clicks to whistles to "Western" vowels and consonants. By the time they are six to eight months old, though, they are only making those sounds that are specific to their mother tongue. In fact, careful tests of young infants reveal that by the time they are four months old, infants can no longer "hear" speech sounds that aren't used in their native languages.

Finally, somewhere between nine to twelve months at the earliest and eighteen months at the latest, most normally developing infants begin uttering their first real words. The sounds are correct, the rhythm and pitch are proper, and the sound clusters (words) are clearly associated with concrete objects or persons. A child whose mother tongue is American English, for example, will say *mama* and know it means Mom, *dada* and know it refers to Daddy, *caa* and associate it with the little furry creature she loves to chase after and hug.

A NATURAL EXPERIMENT

Antonio Damasio has made a career out of following in the footsteps of Broca and Wernicke. He studies people who have been affected by the "natural experiments" of strokes, accidents, and various illnesses that have damaged their brains. He learns what functions these people have lost and uncovers the connections between those lost functions and the damaged parts of their brain. Damasio's major partner in this work has been his wife, Hanna, a world-renowned expert in the use of MRI (magnetic resonance imaging) and PET (positron emission tomography) to map the brain. Together the two Damasios have been able to develop highly precise "functional maps" of the brain's language regions.

One of the people that the two Damasios have worked with for several years is a man they identify as "Boswell." A serious brain disease caused severe damage to several large areas of Boswell's brain. Since then, he has lost much of his ability to identify or recall certain categories of objects and events. His deficiencies are both fascinating and puzzling. For example, if Boswell is shown the appropriate pictures, he can promptly identify furniture, kitchen utensils, and most garden tools. These are all "human-made objects." But he cannot identify most musical instruments, even though they also fall into the "human-made" category. He also has extreme difficulty with some categories of "natural objects." Boswell cannot name fruits with rounded shapes, such as apples, animals of the cat family, or horselike animals. However, he has no trouble identifying bananas, elephants, or giraffes. He can also identify by name any human body part.

Antonio and Hanna Damasio soon discovered a pattern to Boswell's selective linguistic impairments. All of the objects and concepts that Boswell has problems naming are ones denoted by *proper and common nouns*. He has no problems with objects or concepts having to do with attributes, states of being, and relationships. Verbs, prepositions, conjunctions, and adjectives give him no difficulty. Also, his grammar is perfect, so Boswell's brain has not lost its ability to use the basic rules of language formation.

The specific pattern of Boswell's brain damage and associated language problems provide clues to how the brain stores language. For example, Boswell clearly has problems forming concepts and linking them to specific events and entities. The Damasios believe this is linked to the destruction of areas in the middle and frontal regions of his left and right temporal lobes. These areas appear to be a major part of the brain's conceptual subsystem—where the brain creates and stores memories that are what we call concepts. A concept is not so much a word or phrase as a nonverbal form of knowledge. This kind of information resides, among other places, in the middle and frontal parts of the temporal lobes.

Boswell also has some problems forming words and sentences, which has been traced to damage in his brain's left perisylvian cortex, a part of the left cerebral hemisphere that includes areas long known to be associated with language, such as Broca's and Wernicke's areas. But the perisylvian cortex is somewhat broader than just those two language-related regions. The Damasios believe that Boswell's strange problems with certain proper and common nouns is caused by damage both to these regions of his brain and to the neural connections between them and the brain's frontal lobes.

APHASIAS

Aphasia is a language disturbance caused by damage to the brain. It affects a person's ability to speak or write, or to understand spoken or written language.

The leading causes of aphasia are head injury, stroke, brain tumors, and degenerative brain diseases like Alzheimer's disease. (See chapter 11 for more on Alzheimer's.) People with aphasia cannot connect the grammar and symbols of language with the nonverbal knowledge, concepts, and representations that constitute thought. They are unable to translate their nonverbal thoughts and concepts into words and sentences. If a person with aphasia is shown a picture of an apple, for example, she may *know* that it is an apple but be unable to translate that knowledge into the verbal word "apple." The opposite is often also true. That is, an aphasiac often is unable to translate a word or sentence into the appropriate concept. A person with aphasia may be shown the word "apple" written on a piece of paper and then be asked to describe the object the word represents. He or she might reply, "This is a fruit that is red or gold, and round—spherical, actually. Very tasty, sometimes quite sweet and sometimes tart. They make great pies. You can eat them whole and throw away the core, slice 'em up and eat them that way, or peel them. The state of Washington is one of the major places where they're grown." An aphasiac, however, could not provide any such information, since she cannot connect the word "apple" to the nonverbal, mental concepts associated with it.

Aphasia not only involves damage to a person's ability to communicate verbally; it also can impair abilities that rely on "internal speech." This is the ongoing internal monologue inside our heads. Aphasia can severely disrupt creativity, decision making, and the ability to carry out arithmetical calculations.

Several different types of aphasia have been classified. They include:

- Broca's aphasia, also known as expressive, motor, nonfluent, or telegrammatic aphasia. Broca's aphasia comes in two varieties:
- Broca's area aphasia, which occurs when the brain damage occurs only in Broca's area itself or in nearby white matter. This form of aphasia usually causes only temporary damage to language abilities—a condition that is medically referred to as "aphemia."
- True Broca's aphasia, when the damage is to an area of the brain much larger than just Broca's area. People with true Broca's aphasia cannot name things correctly, cannot properly assemble letter-sounds into syllables or proper words, and are unable to correctly repeat sentences.
- Wernicke's aphasia, also called receptive, sensory, fluent, or jargon aphasia. The brain regions damaged include Wernicke's area. Patients with Wernicke's aphasia can speak fluently, but their speech

sounds like nonsensical jargon. They often get the order of sounds and sound clusters mixed up. They appear to have lost the ability to create grammatical speech—language that follows rules of syntax—and have difficulty selecting the right words for their intended meanings.

- Conduction aphasia, involving damage to either a small region in the left cerebral hemisphere, lying above and behind both Broca's and Wernicke's areas, or a part of the brain lying just above Wernicke's area, in the left primary auditory cortex. Also damaged or destroyed are the feedback and feed-forward neural fibers that connect the temporal, parietal, and frontal lobes. These connections are probably part of the neural network that makes it possible for us to combine the basic sounds of words (called phonemes) into syllables and words. People with conduction aphasia can understand essential sentences and can speak intelligently but are unable to combine phonemes correctly and to repeat sentences. They cannot come up with the right words in specific naming tests.

- Global aphasia, which involves damage to many brain areas at once, including Broca's area and Wernicke's area as well as the frontal, temporal, and/or parietal lobes. Global aphasia causes an almost total loss of the ability to both speak and understand language. People with global aphasia cannot speak consciously and deliberately, though they may be able to generate "automatic speech" or "non-deliberate speech." Some people with global aphasia can hum tunes they learned before their brain damage, name the days of the week, or recite childhood verses. But they can comprehend only a few verbs or nouns they may hear.

FRAGMENTS OF LANGUAGE

We've already seen that the brain "takes apart" the visual images that arrive at the primary visual cortex and analyzes each aspect separately. Bits and pieces are stored in different locations. In the same way, the experiences of people suffering from various kinds of aphasia reveal that the brain stores language in the same fashion—in fragments. What's more, it also appears that the brain stores certain kinds of *nonverbal* knowledge in specific regions or neural networks and the words or phrases that correspond to these concepts in *other* storage bins.

This kind of fragmented storage of different parts of language, and of the concepts represented by a word or phrase, is the best explanation available for the often puzzling consequences of strokes and brain injuries. It is not uncommon for stroke victims to be unable to verbally identify an object shown to them, yet still "know" what it is. For example, a person suffering from this kind of brain damage may be shown a coffee cup and asked to name it. He cannot. Perhaps he can identify it as a "round thing," or as "hot." But he cannot, as hard as he may try, conjure up the phrase "coffee cup." Other people with damaged brains have a somewhat different problem. Given a written or spoken word or phrase, they cannot connect it with the proper nonverbal information. Suppose you say to this man, "Coffee cup." He looks at you and shakes his head. "I . . . don't know what you mean." Or you may show him the words "coffee cup" on a computer screen or piece of paper and get a similar response. Perhaps you show this person a piece of paper with the words "coffee cup" written on it and say, "Can you describe this to me?" The man is not able to do it. He may have been drinking four cups of coffee a day for the last forty years, but he cannot describe a coffee cup.

Now suppose a coffee cup is pressed into his hands and he is asked to demonstrate what one does with this object. Without hesitation, he lifts the coffee cup to his lips and pantomimes drinking from it. *He knows what it is; he knows it is a coffee cup*, or at least a cup that is used for drinking. Somewhere in his brain, the knowledge of what a coffee cup is and what it's used for still remains. It is still knowledge that the brain can access and effectively use. But that knowledge *never becomes conscious.*

We assume that our knowledge of the world—of people, places, things, events—is inextricably linked to the words we use to describe them. This is not true. In the world of immediate experience, events and objects do not have labels attached to them saying "father," "Judy," "Marie Celestre's sudden death," "coffee cup." Our experiences of people, places, things, and events are initially nonverbal. This nonverbal information itself does not create either the experience or the feeling of *knowing.* When the connections between language and concepts are broken, a person will find himself or herself lost in a world always a bit out of focus, stumbling through a landscape pockmarked with verbal or conceptual potholes, never quite able to regain balance.

GEORGE OJEMANN AND THE BRAIN'S LANGUAGE REGIONS

More than a century after Broca's and Wernicke's pioneering discoveries, we are beginning to learn that much of what we "knew" about language processing in the brain is wrong. It is indeed true that Broca's area and Wernicke's area play roles in language. However, researchers have also found that the brain creates, stores, and manipulates language in areas far removed from Broca's and Wernicke's. These new insights have come about in part through the creation of new, highly detailed maps of language function in the brain.

One of the people who has created some of these new maps is George Ojemann, a neurosurgeon at the University of Washington in Seattle. His work has in large part followed in the footsteps of Wilder Penfield, the Canadian-American neurosurgeon who was born in Spokane, Washington. The maps that Ojemann creates are a blend of the old and the new. They include not only Broca's and Wernicke's areas but also a whole new pattern of new language sites. Many are in the left cerebral hemisphere, the dominant hemisphere for language. But not all are found there. Taken as a whole, these patterns of language sites Ojemann finds in his patients can be thought of as unique, one-of-a-kind neural tapestries or as a cerebral fingerprint of language.

Ojemann's primary clinical vocation is the surgical treatment of epilepsy. Epilepsy is a brain disorder in which nerve signals "fire" abnormally and cause convulsive seizures. Scar tissue (called lesions) in the brain can provoke some seizures. However, doctors are often unable to determine the reason for many epileptic attacks. If a person has more than one seizure, they are formally called epileptic attacks rather than seizures. About one half of 1 percent of the general population suffers from epileptic attacks. There are three generally recognized types of epileptic attacks: grand mal, petit mal, and infantile. A grand mal attack is usually marked by strongly contracted muscles, physical collapse, and a lapse into unconsciousness. Attacks usually last from two to five minutes and are followed by deep sleep. A petit mal attack usually manifests itself as a loss of awareness for a minute or less. The person often resumes whatever activity she or he was doing without any awareness that something unusual has happened. Children under the age of three sometimes have epileptic attacks which cause them to jackknife their bodies into awkward postures. The electroencephalogram (EEG) is often used to detect areas of irritability in the brain that take place during epileptic attacks. The majority of all people with epilepsy use drugs to effectively treat their condition. Barbital and phenobarbital, for example, have long been used to treat epilepsy because of their anticonvulsant properties.

However, not all cases of epilepsy yield to drugs. Some conditions remain intractable. In these cases, the only solution is to find the precise area of the brain where the "electrical storm" originates and surgically remove or destroy it.

Many of his patients are awake and aware when Ojemann operates on them. Because the brain itself has no pain sensors,* it is possible and often helpful to the surgeon for the patient to be awake during this kind of surgery. The experiments which Ojemann has carried out for more than a decade now have all been done during these operations.

Pinpointing language functions is also only part of the brain mapping that Ojemann has done. All of his experiments in the surgical theater are aimed at investigating how the brain works. They include studies of nondominant brain functions in the nondominant hemisphere, such as spatial functions. Ojemann has also carried out numerous studies that probe memory changes in the brain.

Ojemann and other researchers today have at their disposal a variety of tools to create new maps of language in the brain. One is electrical-stimulation mapping. This technique uses electrical stimulation to specific regions of the brain, applied through tiny electrodes. The researchers then note if any particular function or activity is either triggered or suppressed. Another is the tool used by the Damasios—data that come from a change in the function of a brain area. Sometimes the changes take place as a result of the "natural experiments" studied by the Damasios and others. An area of the brain is damaged, and a change in some cerebral function takes place. These usually include aphasias and other forms of brain damage. If the person has suffered the loss of a specific language ability, this can establish a link between the damaged brain area and the disrupted or lost linguistic function.

Another source of this type of data is electrical stimulation of a cortical region during some kind of brain operation—the kind of work done by American-Canadian neurosurgeon Wilder Penfield, starting in the 1930s. Using a microelectrode to stimulate different parts of a patient's

---

*Though the blood vessels in the brain have pain sensors in them, the neurons themselves do not.

exposed brain, Penfield created temporary changes in specific brain areas and then noted the motor, sensory, or mental function associated with that brain area. Like Ojemann, Penfield carried out his experiments during operations to cure people of epilepsy. He discovered the specific parts of the brain's motor cortex that control the fingers, toes, eyelids, and other body parts. He also found brain areas that stored different sensory memories. One patient might hear a fragment of a melody when one part of his cortex was stimulated. Another might recall the smell of apple pie.

When Ojemann wants to do a language map, he also uses MRI and PET scans. These provide him with detailed functional maps of the brain while the patient carries out specific language activities. He can then match them with the patient's performance on language tests made during the surgery and the experiment.

Ojemann uses several different electrical recording techniques. One is a computerized version of the venerable EEG. In recent years computer technology has greatly enhanced the amount and quality of data researchers can acquire using EEGs. In particular, computerized EEGs can detect *evoked potentials*. These minuscule changes in voltage occur when the brain responds to specific stimuli. By filtering out the background noise of the brain, sophisticated computer programs allow the researcher to detect these minute changes in brain waves. Neuroscientists also use evoked potential EEGs to study stroke victims, people with brain tumors and multiple sclerosis, and the brain activity of newborn infants.

An EEG reading, even a sophisticated one of evoked potentials, is a passive recording of the brain's ongoing electrical activity, often in response to specific tasks or actions. Electrical stimulation is an active process. As noted earlier, a researcher uses tiny electrical impulses applied through microelectrodes to stimulate a part of the brain. The researcher then uses other techniques, such as PET or MRI or EEG, to track the brain's responses.

Ojemann also uses a new variation of the EEG technique called electrocorticography, or ECoG, an extremely sophisticated and delicate technique for recording the electrical activity of individual neurons in the brain. Using ECoG, Ojemann can find the precise areas in the person's temporal lobe that are damaged, or misfiring, and are causing the epileptic attacks. Once he's found those regions, he can cut it out of the brain with minimal damage to surrounding areas.

All these experiments, by the way, are done with the patient's consent. Ojemann gets it in writing before the operation, confirms it verbally just before entering the operating room, and checks with the conscious patient one more time before the experiment actually starts. The person can back out at any time. Sometimes a patient does just that. When that happens, no experiments take place, and Ojemann simply proceeds with the operation to stop the epileptic attacks.

Using a local anesthesia so that the patient remains conscious, Ojemann first drills a small hole in the skull. Then using a specialized device that includes a hydraulic micromanipulator, he lowers a tungsten electrode less than 5 microns in diameter into the brain itself. Ojemann locates a neuron, or small neuron cluster, in the area to be tested. Once its electrical output has remained stable for several minutes, he begins the testing process. Each electrical recording takes from fifteen to thirty minutes. The patient, fully conscious, lies on one side with his or her head in a padded headrest. The patient obviously cannot see the operation itself but can see and talk with the people who are carrying out the tests. Ojemann and his team provide the patient with particular stimuli or tasks to carry out. For language mapping, these may include reading specific words or phrases, listening to words or phrases or to musical passages, or thinking silently about a particular word or phrase.

With this kind of probing and mapping, Ojemann has uncovered a hitherto unsuspected aspect of language in the brain. You could call them "language fingerprints."

LANGUAGE'S NEURAL FINGERPRINTS

Neuroscientists have long had a standard model for the brain's language organization. In this model, language processing in the brain begins in Wernicke's area, in the posterior temporal cortex. Here the brain decodes basic language concepts. Next, Broca's area, on the left rear edge of the brain's frontal lobe, takes over, modulating the motor expression of spoken language.

However, researchers have found that the brain actually processes language in much the same way it handles visual, auditory, and other sensory inputs: in tiny pieces. Language function is fragmented, and there are many more fragments and therefore language sites in the brain than most brain researchers had ever realized. With his meticulous micorelectrode recordings of electrical activity of neurons, George

Ojemann has discovered the existence of previously unsuspected language sites. Each consists of clumps of neurons about the size of a marble. Each clump of neurons appears to specialize in a particular language function, says Ojemann. One patch of neurons may deal with a specific rule of grammar, while another recalls verbs. Still another clump processes words from a second or third language (English, say, instead of Hungarian). Another recalls nouns or pronouns in the person's mother tongue.

In well over 90 percent of all people the bulk of the brain's language regions are in the left cerebral hemisphere. In most of the people Ojemann has studied, the great majority of the marble-sized language compartments are indeed found in the left temporal and parietal lobes—most but by no means all. A significant number are also in the right hemisphere. Language still turns out to be highly lateralized; it's just not as "left brain" a process as has long been assumed.

Much more surprising is another discovery by Ojemann. The language nodes in a person's dominant hemisphere turn out to be "individually localized." Their physical arrangement differs from person to person. In fact, they appear to be unique for each individual. Call them neural fingerprints for language if you wish. It turns out that we each have a unique arrangement of neurons and neural networks for language ability.

Why the unique, individualized nature of the brain's language organization? No one really knows, but Ojemann has suggested some possible reasons. First, each of our brains as a whole is physically unique. Each human brain has a slightly different pattern to its cerebral folds and fissures and to the physical location of each lobe. These kinds of differences are likely caused by small differences in each person's genetic code. The coding in our DNA provides the directions for the development of the brain's shape and structure. Each of us has tiny variations in our genetic code. These variations account for the unique patterns of ridges and fissures, just as they account for our unique fingerprints.

However, Ojemann thinks that genetic differences are not entirely responsible for the individual patterns of the brain's many language patches. Environment and experiences must also play a role. As we've already seen, the infant human brain is incredibly malleable and is programmed from birth to respond to the environment. Each sensory experience molds the brain's structure. Each brain responds to its particular set of experiences and weaves a neural tapestry slightly different from every other one. And these unique neural language fingerprints develop very early in life. George Ojemann's brain-mapping experiments have shown that the distribution of language areas in children from ages four to ten is as individual as it is in adults.

LANGUAGE CONVERGENCE ZONES

Ojemann has used his expertise in neurosurgery as a way to map the brain's language centers. Meanwhile, Hanna and Antonio Damasio and their colleagues have been working with their brain-damaged patients and doing the same. Like those of Ojemann, the Damasios' findings both confirm some long-held beliefs about linguistic organization in the brain and add new discoveries.

For example, the Damasios have added their own confirmation of the brain's language laterality. They have found that the front part of the left temporal cortex is dedicated to language. Specifically, this particular language region lies along the front and bottom of the left temporal lobe. The corresponding area in the right temporal lobe plays no role at all in language. If it is damaged by a stroke, for example, the person will not lose any language ability. The same is not true for the region in the left temporal lobe.

If this particular part of the temporal lobe is damaged by a stroke or accident, a person will be unable to retrieve information about certain entities. Damasio defines an "entity" as a person or thing. For example, a person with scar tissue in this part of his brain might not be able to access the name of a specific individual, like Elizabeth Taylor. He may also be unable to call up the common nouns for nonunique categories of animals or objects, such as "porcupine" or "bridge." For some reason, damage to the front and bottom parts of the left temporal lobe cuts a person off from the collection of words that denote concrete entities and actions.

A person's actual knowledge of these entities is unaffected. If you ask such a person, "What's a porcupine?" he can tell you that it's an animal covered with quills. If you show him a picture of Elizabeth Taylor, he can tell you that she's a famous actress who starred in *National Velvet* when she was a child, that she's been married many times, and that she has beautiful violet eyes.

When another part of the left temporal is damaged, a person will be unable to retrieve proper nouns—and only proper nouns. She cannot call up "Mount Rainier," or "Ventura," or "John Guth."

Ojemann has made similar findings during his own mapping studies of living human brains. He has found that specific neurons or neuron clusters in our brains deal with particular language tasks. This also holds true for second and third languages. A person who speaks both English and Spanish will have a specific language area for, say, naming objects in English and another one for naming objects in Spanish. That includes a specific area for naming objects in American sign language. Many of these language neurons and neuron clusters are found in the right hemisphere as well as the left. Thus, it's clear from the work of both Ojemann and the Damasios that the brain deals with language in a piecemeal fashion.

To explain how the brain pulls together the different parts of a word, plus the grammatical rules for forming sentences, Antonio Damasio has proposed his "convergence zone" theory. The brain, he says, does not have specific regions for storing particular concepts like "white coffee cup." Instead, the brain stores the concept as a set of attributes, each in different locations. "White" is in one region, "cup shape" in another, a particular texture (a touch input) somewhere else, and so on. We know this to be true from the kinds of dysfunctions people suffer when they have strokes. Remember the woman who lost all ability to see color— even the ability to imagine color. For her there is no longer any such thing as a white coffee cup. So when a person thinks of a white coffee cup, the brain activates the different storage areas and brings all those attributes together to form a white coffee cup. Thus, the concept "white coffee cup" never exists in some particular spatial location in the brain. The concept itself exists only *in time*, at those moments during which the brain is combining all the fragmentary aspects together.

Damasio believes the same process goes on with language. His favorite example is the one just used, the coffee cup. The word cup is made of three language sounds or phonemes. Linguists write them as /k/, /ə/, and /p/. Different neuron clusters store these specific phonemes. When a person says "cup," the brain pulls together these phonemes from their storage areas and combines them into the word.

The question is, how does the brain know to correctly combine concept fragments into concepts or sounds into words? Damasio thinks this is done by other clusters of neurons he calls *convergence zones*. These tiny brain regions store the "codes," or instructions, needed to properly combine /k/, /ə/, and /p/ into "cup," or "white," "crushable," "texture," "cone shape," into "white coffee cup." When a person suffers a stroke and loses her ability to name specific people like Elizabeth Taylor, either a particular convergence zone has been damaged, or its connections to language and concept storage areas are broken.

Ojemann's microelectrical probes of the brain have revealed some intriguing supporting evidence for this theory. The different parts of the brain's language systems, Ojemann says, seem to operate in parallel rather than in a linear fashion. Instead of processing language one step at a time, the brain appears to carry out several processes simultaneously. This would seem to offer support for the existence of convergence zones. Different areas of the brain take care of different components of language: naming, verbal memory, grammar, storage of specific phonemes. The brain activates the necessary regions nearly simultaneously. The result: there is no one physical location in the brain where "language happens." The different pieces of language are stored in different places. But we learn, comprehend, and create spoken or signed language *in time*, as the brain brings all the pieces together moment by moment. Only something like Antonio Damasio's convergence zones can actually make this kind of scheme work.

BRAINS AND GENDER

Women's brains are in general smaller in size than those of men. This is directly connected to the simple fact that human females are generally somewhat smaller than human males.* However, in recent years several studies using PET and MRI have begun finding actual *functional* differences between the brains of men and women. One such difference has to do with language.

Sally Shaywitz was one of the principle investigators in some of this research. A behavioral scientist at Yale University, Shaywitz and her colleagues were using functional MRI (abbreviated fMRI) to study the brain basis of reading disorders. They began, as all such studies must, by getting MRI scans of people who were normal readers. Shaywitz and her husband, Bennett Shaywitz, a neurobiologist, used a rhyming test. The subjects were nineteen men and nineteen women. As they lay in the MRI scanner, each was asked to read a series of nonsense words and determine if they rhymed. The words might be something like "lete" and "jete," or perhaps "feepo" and "sneepo."† In order to determine if

---

*In scientific terms, this is known as sexual dimorphism. Though real in humans, it is not nearly as pronounced as it is in many other species of animals, including other primates.
†You've just done the test, haven't you? Did they rhyme? How did you find out?

these nonsense words rhyme, the volunteers had to mentally "sound them out" or say them silently. In order to do *that*, they had to use phonemes. Phonemes are the basic sounds, the essential building blocks, of a language. All this was to establish a "baseline" for the next part of the experiments—fMRI scans of the brains of people who suffered from reading difficulties such as dyslexia.

But when the Shaywitzes and their colleagues examined the fMRI brain scans of the normal subjects, they discovered something surprising. They found actual functional differences between the way men's and women's brains processed this reading skill. All nineteen men and nineteen women used a small area of brain tissue lying near Broca's area in the left cerebral hemisphere. However, eleven of the women *also* used a comparable region located in the *right* cerebral hemisphere.

Shaywitzes' findings is the first definitive proof that women use their brains differently than men to perform the same task with the same results. And it is a clear indication that the brains of women may not be as "lateralized" as those of men. "The brain," Sally Shaywitz has said, "is a lot more complicated than we thought." It's now clear that it "has lots of different ways to get to the same result." What was particularly intriguing to her is that this difference has to do with reading. Reading is not a basic survival skill, nor does it provide its practitioners with better reproductive advantages. There's no evolutionary reason for the brain to develop different modes for doing reading. This skill involves thinking, cognition, and yet the brains of women have found ways of doing it that are different from those used by males and just as effective.

WATCHING THE BRAIN READ

No one has yet actually found the Damasios' convergence zones, though Ojemann's marble-sized language regions definitely exist. However, several researchers have been busy making PET and MRI maps of the brain's language regions on a somewhat larger scale. The most impressive such maps by far have come from the laboratory of Steven Petersen at Washington University in St. Louis. A close colleague of Marcus Raichle, Petersen has made impressive use of PET to reveal the brain at work as it speaks and reads.

In one well-documented experiment Petersen and his colleagues wanted to answer an old question about reading. Most children are at least four years old before they begin mastering the most basic reading skills. This is obviously related to the brain's own physical and structural development, though environmental factors may also play a role. Once a person learns to read, though, the brain can almost instantly recognize whether or not a string of letters is a word. Does the brain do this by recognizing the shape of the word itself or by checking the spelling?

Petersen worked with eight healthy adults who possessed normal reading skills. First, they took PET scans of the volunteers' brains as they stared at a blank computer screen. This provided the baseline brain PET images for later comparison. Next, the researchers did PET scans of the subjects as they read items on the computer screen from four different lists. Each computerized list contained 256 different words or stimuli. One list consisted of common nouns, such as "cat," "board," and "light." A second list was made up of pseudowords, such as "floop" or "tweal," strings of letters that look and sound like real words because they follow standard English rules of spelling. A third list contained nothing but strings of consonants, such as "jvjfc" or "nlpfz." The fourth list was a set of meaningless straight and curved lines with no correspondence to any English letters. One word or stimulus per second appeared on the computer screen and remained there for .15 second. After an .85 second pause the next stimulus would appear.

By using the PET computer software to subtract the baseline image from the other images, Petersen and his associates were able to see exactly which areas in the brain were active for each of the four kinds of reading stimuli. The results were intriguing.

When the subjects silently read the real common noun ("light") and the pseudoword ("floop"), a region of the brain called the left medial extrastriate visual cortex became very active. This region lies outside of, but close to, the primary visual cortex.* According to Petersen, this region appears to distinguish strings of letters that do or do not follow standard English spelling rules. This clearly takes place early in the visual processing task and is one of the first steps the brain takes to read a word.

LEFT EQUALS LANGUAGE

In nearly everyone, language functions are concentrated in the brain's

---

*The primary visual cortex is sometimes called the striate cortex because its highly organized structure looks like a series of striations or lines under a microscope. Areas near this region are thus called "extrastriate."

left hemisphere. They are lateralized. Most sensory and motor functions are bilateral, or spread around through both the left and right cerebral hemispheres. In the case of language, however, the left hemisphere appears to rule. Why this is the case remains something of a mystery. One of George Ojemann's colleagues (and his occasional coauthor), neurophysiologist and award-winning author William Calvin of the University of Washington, has offered a speculative but intriguing theory. He calls it "the throwing Madonna" hypothesis.

Calvin argues that the development of verbal language and its concentration in the left cerebral hemisphere is directly tied to the way early human mothers held their babies, right-handedness, and the way they threw rocks. Briefly, it goes like this:

1. Most early human moms (Calvin hypothesizes) held their infants in their *left arms*, thus putting the baby's head and ears close to Mom's heart. Babies who hear Mom's heartbeat are more relaxed and secure than those who don't hear Mom's heart as clearly, because their heads lie near Mom's right breast.

2. In any case, this left Mom's right hand free to do all kinds of things: pick fruit from trees, berries from bushes, roots from the ground. It also freed Mom's right hand to pick up rocks.

3. Why rocks? Well, a nice-sized rock, thrown accurately, can kill a rabbit at many paces. This in turn gave the brain's *left hemisphere* (which governs the body's right side; ergo, the right hand and arm) plenty of opportunities to learn and remember how to accurately throw rocks. Not only are the mathematical calculations involved in accurately aiming and throwing a rock pretty complex; so is the timing. In fact, the timing of throwing a rock accurately enough and consistently enough to increase survival chances involves a certain amount of anticipation. You have to "lead" the target; you have to make an educated guess; you have to project events into the near future.

4. This consistent and persistent use of certain areas in the left cerebral hemisphere would likely lead to a marked propensity to right-handedness in humans. The moms most likely to survive would presumably be the ones who could, among other things, consistently hit a rabbit at many paces throwing right-handed. These were the moms with brains genetically predisposed to more efficient learning of eye-hand coordination in the left hemisphere.

They tended to make more babies who survived into adulthood to become moms who also had a propensity for right-handedness; and so it goes.

5. This highly complex use of muscle groups could also come in handy for, and perhaps even lead to, the complex control of the muscles needed to create verbal speech. What's more, the ability to intuit the location of a rabbit at many paces and then hit it with one well-aimed rock could also help develop cognitive abilities. And those abilities could lead to the development of the method of communication we call language.

6. Finally, this all leads to a lateralization of language functions in the left hemisphere—not for any grand or mysterious reason but simply as a side effect of humanity's programming for right-handedness. One might say that language and rock throwing go hand in hand, but that would be a truly terrible pun.

This summary probably does not do justice to either Calvin's hypothesis or his lucid and entertaining writing. His own books do a much better job of explaining the concept of "the throwing Madonna," including the one of that title.*

IT'S IN THE TIMING

While William Calvin's "throwing Madonna" theory for language lateralization is intriguing, it is certainly not the only one. In fact, a researcher at Rutgers University has one that's just as attention getting. Better yet, it's testable.

Paula Tallal works at the University's Center for Molecular and Behavioral Neuroscience. For more than twenty years now she has studied children with developmental dysphasia, a language impairment, and dyslexia, a reading dysfunction. Children with these dysfunctions have difficulty both hearing and forming the subtle differences between and among speech sounds. That in turn means they suffer delays in language development and in learning to read. And that leads to all kinds of learning, behavioral, and social-skills problems later in life.

---

*Calvin, William H. *The Throwing Madonna: Essays on the Brain* (New York: McGraw-Hill, 1983, 1991). Though now out of print in the United States, *The Throwing Madonna* can still be found in many libraries and used bookstores or ordered from the University Bookstore in Seattle.

Suppose I say the following phonemes or speech sounds aloud, one after another, rapidly: *pa ba*. It sounds more like *paba*. Most of you will effortlessly distinguish the two sounds. Most children can do so, too. But children with developmental dysphasia cannot. They might hear *papa* or *baba* but not *paba*. Nor is the problem limited just to sounds. A more basic impairment is involved. The brains of these children apparently cannot process two sensory signals that arrive in rapid succession. Normally developing children can distinguish between two 75-millisecond-long sounds that have only an 8 millisecond break between them. Children with dysphasia need a break of at least 300 milliseconds—37.5 times as long—in order to distinguish the two tones from one another. These same children also cannot distinguish between two rapid taps on their skin. To them, it does not feel like two finger taps, but one. As Tallal has said, "If you have to do it in tens of milliseconds, these kids can't do it."

This is a problem in real life. Because, in real life, most phonemes change rapidly as the mouth, tongue, and lips move in spoken language. Those changes in phonemes take place on an average of once every 40 milliseconds. This doesn't mean that you use as many as twenty-five different speech sounds in one second. It means that, on the average, the change from one phoneme to the next takes place in about four-hundredths of a second. Most children have no problem with that, Tallal found in tests using the computer-generated sounds *da* and *ba* that changed frequency every 40 milliseconds. Children with dysphasia do. Only when she extended the time to 80 milliseconds could the language-impaired children distinguish the sounds *da* and *ba*.

One well-known hint that the left hemisphere is dominant for language is what scientists call "the right-ear advantage." If a person simultaneously hears different phonemes in each ear, he or she will more accurately perceive the phoneme presented to the right ear. The right ear's auditory nerves are primarily wired to the left cerebral hemisphere. Tallal and her colleagues put the right-ear advantage to the test. They had a group of subjects simultaneously listen with both ears to two different computer-generated speech sounds, such as *ba* and *da*. At first, the speech sounds changed every 40 milliseconds. Sure enough, the subjects could perceive the sounds heard with their right ears more readily than those presented to their left ears. Then Tallal extended the time between frequency changes to 80 milliseconds. The right-ear advantage disappeared. Tallal concluded that it wasn't the information itself that the left hemisphere was looking for but the *duration* for which the information was presented.

Tallal then tied this "temporal processing" of speech sounds to the left hemisphere in another series of tests. These were done with adults who had suffered stroke damage. She presented two groups of patients with computer-generated tones in two-beep sequences. One group, the control group, had suffered brain damage to their right hemispheres. These people could easily distinguish between the two sounds, even when the intervals between them was as short as 8 milliseconds. By contrast, the group who had suffered damage to their left hemispheres could not distinguish between the tones until at least a 300-millisecond interval separated them. They needed almost forty times as much time between the sounds to tell them apart. This strongly suggests, says Tallal, that the left hemisphere is specialized for processing rapid changes in sound signals.

Tallal has worked with Steve Petersen and Marcus Raichle to pin down the exact area in the brain that may be involved with this. Along with them and their coworker Julie Fiez, Tallal used PET scans to map the brain activity of a group of people taking a special hearing test. The subjects listened to four sets of sounds. Some included rapid changes from sound to sound, and others did not. Some also had verbal meaning, while others did not. The researchers found a specific region in the left frontal lobe that lit up only when the set of stimuli included sounds that changed rapidly from one to the next. It didn't matter if the sounds were actual words or just sound patterns. This particular brain region did not become active when vowel sounds were used. Vowel sounds have a constant frequency—*ayyyyy*, *eeeee*, and so on. This area only activated when the input consisted of sounds that changed rapidly. Finally, it turns out that when this brain region is damaged by strokes or injuries, aphasia almost always results.

Tallal and her colleagues think that this connection between the left hemisphere and rapid signal analysis may allow us to make the evolutionary connection between language in humans and other forms of animal communication. For example, just how far back, evolutionarily speaking, does this right-ear advantage extend? Tallal and her colleagues have done experiments with rats, using (believe it or not) tiny headphones to let them simultaneously hear different tones in each ear.

Yes, rats have a strong right-ear advantage, which means their tiny left hemispheres are specialized for detecting and processing rapid signal changes. Rats are probably many tens of millions of years older, evo-lutionarily speaking, than humans. It should come as no surprise, then, that our prehuman ancestors just a few million years ago pushed this left-hemisphere specialization just a little bit further.

THE WORK by Paula Tallal reveals a provocative and powerful connec-tion between humans and other animals and between language and the brain's left hemisphere. And it is one that rings true when taken togeth-er with so much else we have learned about the brain. For example, it suggests that Damasio's language convergence zones are real and work as he suggests: tying language fragments together *in time* rather than in some physical location in space, in the brain.

And it also fits well with the many other discoveries made using MRI, PET, CT scans, and even EEG, the discoveries that reveal the brain to be modular in nature. The human brain is not some monolith-ic meat computer that processes data in a linear, one-piece-at-a-time fashion. The brain is made up of thousands of different modules or sub-systems. Its myriad of neural networks constantly swap information back and forth, probably guided by rules or "codes" contained in still other tiny neuron modules.

Finally, Paula Tallal's discoveries also give us a glimpse into how truly strange the brain really is. Think about it for a moment. That con-versation you had earlier today with your coworker, your friend, your lover? Despite the *uhs* and *mms* and "y'knows," it was a pretty smooth and actually seamless stream of language. Right? Yes, and no. Your actu-al speech was. Behind it, though, flashing millisecond by millisecond through multitrillion synaptic pathways, your brain was creating your verbal speech word by word from widely distributed fragments of sound memories.

When we look closely at language, we discover it's not seamless at all. The seamlessness of speech is an illusion, one created by the very organ that makes it possible for us to perceive "reality": the brain.

What else is an illusion?

CHAPTER 11

BREAKDOWNS

My MOTHER sometimes jokes about Alzheimer's disease. This usually happens when she forgets something. "Ohhhhh, boy," she says, smiling and shaking her head. "I must be coming down with Alzheimer's." Or, "Listen, if I end up with Alzheimer's, just *take* me out and *shoot* me!"

My mother is seventy years old. She is still quite spry and as intellectually sharp as she was more than fifty years ago, when her looks and intelligence utterly captivated my father. Does she suffer some short-term memory loss? I suspect so. That's a not uncommon, normal consequence of the aging process. To the best of her knowlege, no one in her family has suffered from this terrible neurological disease. If Mom really does have Alzheimer's, she's sure got her doctor and her family fooled.

However, our family is no stranger to the consequences of brain malfunctions. My father is the oldest of four children. His only brother died of polio right after World War II. His sister Carolyn is alive and well, the mother of two adult sons, and still happily married to her first and only husband. But his other sister, my aunt Joan, was in and out of mental hospitals and halfway houses most of her adult life, sometimes taking her "meds" but more often living a life filled with pain, loneliness, frustration, and fear. She saw things that weren't there, heard voices that no one else discerned. When she died of cancer a few years ago, Dad and Aunt Carolyn were sad but also relieved. Not so much for themselves, though they both had experienced decades of heartbreak, but for Joan herself.

Joan suffered from schizophrenia. My grandmother Augusta Farkas had Parkinson's disease in the last two years before her death. Lulu

Boyd, my great-grandmother, suffered a series of strokes before her death at age ninety-three.

What these tragic medical conditions have in common is the brain. All are brain breakdowns of one kind or another. They also have something else in common: These and several other brain disorders are giving us valuable clues to the nature of the human mind.

As with any other organ of the body, the brain is susceptible to a wide range of disorders. These include the damage to neural tissue from a stroke, when the blood flow to the brain is suddenly reduced or momentarily blocked; tumors, or abnormal masses in the brain; different kinds of infections, such as meningitis; and various traumatic injuries, such as blows to the head. Several diseases are specific to the brain. Epilepsy is caused by abnormal electrical discharges in the brain. As we've seen earlier, its symptoms range from brief lapses in awareness to sudden losses of consciousness, with generalized convulsions. Parkinson's disease, Alzheimer's disease, and Huntington's disease are all devastating disorders that involve specific damage to the brain.

Researchers around the world are searching for treatments and cures for these devastating neurological diseases and conditions. At the same time, these and other researchers are using the new imaging technologies to probe the living brains of volunteers with these disorders. They do so to learn which parts of the brain are involved in each disorder, to learn how different parts of the brain may be simultaneously affected, and to provide other researchers with clues that can lead to treatments and cures.

In the process, the new brain-imaging machines are giving scientists a remarkable—and at times controversial—look at the very nature of consciousness, self-awareness, and the mind.

THE EROSION OF THE MIND

My mother jokes about Alzheimer's because she fears it—a pretty normal way of dealing with fear. We psychologically distance ourselves from it by making fun of it. But Alzheimer's disease is no laughing matter. Its symptoms were long dismissed as normal consequences of human aging, but by the 1980s the medical community recognized it as the most common cause of *dementia* in middle-aged and elderly people. Dementia is a collection of symptoms—or a syndrome—most dramatically characterized by serious declines in social and intellectual abilities.

These changes become so severe that the individual can no longer function as a whole person in daily life. Alzheimer's disease is the major
cause of presenile dementia, dementia not associated with advanced
age. It is also the largest single cause of an advanced degree of brain
impairment known as senile dementia. About 50–60 percent of all cases
of dementia in the United States are caused by Alzheimer's. Former
president Ronald Reagan is just one of the 2.5 to 2.8 million Americans
with this disease. It is extremely rare in young adults and very uncommon among middle-aged people. It occurs in about 4 percent of people
between sixty-five to seventy-four years old, 10 percent of those
between seventy-five and eighty-four years old, and 17 percent of those
aged eighty-five or older.

Some forms of dementia are caused by specific illnesses or neurological conditions and may be treatable to some degree. Alzheimer's disease, the most common cause of dementia, has as yet no known cause
or cure. The symptoms of Alzheimer's include speech disturbances, dis-
orientation, difficulty with abstract thinking, and severe short-term
memory loss. The normal aging process usually involves slight losses of
recent memory, but not the dramatic memory losses associated with
Alzheimer's. These effects eventually lead to the progressive loss of
nearly all major mental faculties. A person with Alzheimer's disease usually remains physically healthy, alert, intelligent, and self-aware until the
later stages of the disease. All the while the personality slowly but irre-
versibly disintegrates. And that, of course, is the true horror of
Alzheimer's. The victim may often *know* that something terrible is happening. Worse, she or he may even know *what* is happening. But to no
avail. The marvelously complex and unique tapestry of behavior and
memories that we call the personality has unraveled.

The causes of Alzheimer's disease are unknown, but we do know that
it is associated with two striking abnormalities in the cellular structure of
brain tissue: neuritic plaques and neurofibrillary tangles. Alzheimer's is
characterized by the death of nerve cells in the cerebral cortex. In 1906
the German neurologist Alois Alzheimer first described the characteristic features of brain cells in people with this condition, and the disease
now bears his name. Victims of the disease also have a deficiency of a
neurotransmitter, or brain chemical, called acetylcholine. This chemical
is vital for communication between brain cells. Some research suggests
the existence of a viruslike causative agent called a *prion*. Other studies
have implicated abnormal concentrations of aluminum in the brain tis-

sue. Neither hypothesis has been proved; indeed, many reputable studies have totally contradicted both of these hypotheses.

More firmly grounded in scientific data is a genetic component. In the late 1980s some researchers believed they had found evidence linking Alzheimer's with the hereditary condition known as Down syndrome. In late 1993 a team of researchers at Duke University Medical Center in Durham, North Carolina, found a much more solid genetic connection. They were able to demonstrate a significant statistical link between Alzheimer's and a gene known as apolipoprotein E-4, often abbreviated apoE-4. This gene is found on the human chromosome known as chromosome 14.

Many of our genes come in different varieties. Just as there can be many different kinds of apples, oranges, and plums, each with different colors and flavors, many of our genes come in different varieties. Geneticists call these variant genes *alleles*. These alleles are usually not defective; they're just slightly different in their chemical composition. In somewhat the same way, a Granny Smith is no more a defective apple than is a Golden Delicious. They're just apples with different colors and flavors.

Genes lie along chromosomes like beads on a string, and the twenty-three chromosomes in the human genetic code come in pairs, for a total of forty-six chromosomes. Thus, we all carry two copies of each gene. These paired copies need not be identical. We can have a Granny Smith apple gene and a Golden Delicious apple gene paired together without any harm, since most gene variants are not really defective. As long as the paired genes do their job—coding for the creation of the right kind of protein—we never notice their differences (table 11.1).

However, some alleles *are* defective. If it's just one of the pair, it may not matter. The normal allele produces the proper protein. If both alleles are defective, though, it can mean real trouble. The apoE gene has several alleles, all denoted by numbers; thus, apoE-4 is the fourth variant of the apoE gene.

One must be careful about leaping to conclusions. Like the drunken swimmer who often doesn't look before leaping, only to find the swimming pool drained, it can be dangerous to one's intellectual health to conclude that apoE-4 *causes* Alzheimer's. It probably doesn't. As any reputable geneticist will tell you, the genes that make up the human genetic code (or genome) and each individual's genetic code don't really cause anything at all. A gene is nothing more than the molecular

Possible Alzheimer's Genes

Chromosome	Age of Onset	% cases: Familial	% cases: All	Protein product
19	60+		40–50%	ApoE4
14	30–60	70–80%		S182
21	45–65	2–3%	< 1%	amyloid precursor protein
?	40–70	–20%	2–3%	?

TABLE 11.1   *Note*: Researchers have tentatively identified as many as four different genes that may play a role in Alzheimer's disease.

instructions for making a protein. It's the *proteins* that do things: detect light in the eye's rod and cone cells, for example, help metabolize sugar, or add a tint of color to our skins. Good evidence now exists for some kind of connection between Alzheimer's and the apoE-4 gene, but what that connection really is remains a mystery. Perhaps the protein created by the gene interrupts the actions of other proteins that control how brain cells grow. That would explain the existence of the neuronal plaques and tangles in the brains of Alzheimer's patients. The consequent breakdown in the brain's structural integrity might then be the proximate cause of Alzheimer's. Or perhaps that's not it at all. Maybe the connection between Alzheimer's and the presence of the apoE-4 gene is not directly causative. Perhaps this particular gene is one of only several that must be present and activated in order to cause Alzheimer's. No one really knows.

One of the particularly vicious aspects of Alzheimer's has been the extreme difficulty in actually diagnosing the disease. Until recently, the only single test that could do so was an autopsy, or brain biopsy, and by then the person is dead. These postmortem exams clearly show the neuritic plaques and neurofibrillary tangles and the significant loss of neurons in the cerebral cortex. Many of the symptoms of Alzheimer's, such as memory loss, can also occur as part of diseases like depression, adverse reaction to prescription drugs, a poorly functioning thyroid, or vitamin B_{12} deficiency. Some of these conditions respond well to treatment, and so a person who is suffering such symptoms needs to have a thorough medical checkup. Alzheimer's may well not be the cause of such symptoms. In the end, the best way to diagnose Alzheimer's in a living person has been to eliminate all other possible causes of the symptoms.

Now, though, the new imaging technologies give researchers and doctors the ability to look at the living brain at work inside the skull. And this new technological vision of brain function is now sharp enough to detect the telltale signs of Alzheimer's. Early in 1995 a group of researchers led by Gary Small of the University of California at Los Angeles used positron-emission tomography (PET) to detect subtle changes in brain function that may well presage the onset of Alzheimer's disease in people who are genetically at risk for the disease.

Small and his colleagues were well aware of Alzheimer's likely genetic connection. And they knew about the Duke University Medical Center findings. They used that to their advantage. First, they recruited thirty-one men and women aged fifty or older who came from families with a history of Alzheimer's. All thirty-one volunteers admitted to experiencing some mild short-term memory problems, such as forgetting where they had placed familiar objects, like car keys or a favorite coffee cup. Other than that, however, they performed quite normally on standard tests of cognitive function. Small then carried out PET scans of the volunteers' brains.

PET scans of people who are already exhibiting all the symptoms of Alzheimer's reveal a distinctive pattern of lowered brain activity. The pattern begins in the area of the brain's cerebral cortex known as the parietal lobe, the region known to be associated with memory, language, and other functions that Alzheimer's damages and finally destroys. However, no one had yet been able to show that PET scans could detect brain-function changes in healthy people who *later* succumbed to Alzheimer's disease. That's where the genetic link to Alzheimer's entered the mix. Small and his team collected blood samples from their thirty-one volunteers and had them tested for the presence of the apoE-4 gene. Twelve of the volunteers had, in fact, inherited the gene. Next, Small's group ran PET scans on the brains of each of the thirty-one men and women in their test group. As we've seen, PET scans measure the brain's use of glucose, a major source of nourishment for neurons. Then the team combined the brain scans and the genetic testing results.

The result was a potential breakthrough in our ability to identify people at high risk of later suffering from Alzheimer's. Of the twelve volunteers who carried the apoE-4 gene, PET scans showed all had significantly reduced metabolism in their brains' parietal regions when compared to the other nineteen who did not carry apoE-4. It appears that in these twelve volunteers, many of the neurons in the brain's parietal lobe were already either dead or working poorly. Though they show no symptoms of any form of dementia, including Alzheimer's, these men and women may already be silently on the road to tragedy.

Until very recently, Small's findings were still preliminary. In early 1996, however, other researchers essentially duplicated Small's results. PET scans have proved to be an effective method of detecting the earliest signs of Alzheimer's, even before any obvious symptoms appear.

They also provide corporations and the medical community with a significant ethical dilemma. It is now possible to tell people that they may have Alzheimer's decades before their minds begin to erode away. But "may" does not necessarily equal "will." A persuasive case can be made that it is unethical to tell people they have a disease that will rob them of every vestige of humanity when no cure or treatment exists for that condition. Every known religion and spiritual path considers the deliberate doing of harm to others as a sin. Providing information per se is neither harmful nor evil, but what if the consequences of that act are overwhelmingly painful? Every diagnosis has consequences. The psychological suffering resulting from an early diagnosis of Alzheimer's might well be overwhelming for most people. Despite what appears to be the prevailing popular opinion, we all bear some measure of ethical and moral responsibility for our actions. Of course, many corporations and individuals stand to make a lot of money by commercializing the availability of an early Alzheimer's diagnosis. To which some might respond with the words of a certain Jewish carpenter of two millennia ago about the impossibility of worshiping both God and money.

Nevertheless, these findings need not be a sentence to premature hopelessness and despair. Researchers around the world are working hard to find both a treatment and a cure for Alzheimer's. The ability to identify people who are in the earliest stages of the disease is in a real sense a hopeful step. With many diseases, such as breast cancer, early detection increases the chances of curing it or starting treatments that can add years of productive and happy life. At this stage in the battle against Alzheimer's, researchers need people who can effectively participate in trials of experimental treatments or cures. Small's work, if confirmed, will be of inestimable value in finally defeating this dreaded brain breakdown.

ALZHEIMER'S AND MAGNETIC RESONANCE IMAGING (MRI)

On the other side of the country another team of researchers has used a different brain-imaging machine to shed light on a different aspect of the Alzheimer's mystery. McLean Hospital is a collection of campuslike brick buildings sitting on a hill in Belmont, Massachusetts. An affiliate of the Harvard Medical School in nearby Boston, McLean is the site of some exciting research on Alzheimer's and other incapacitating brain breakdowns. Bruce Cohen, senior vice president for research at the hospital, has led a team of scientists that has uncovered new information about Alzheimer's that could be crucial in the development of an effective treatment for the disease.

Researchers have long recognized two general types of Alzheimer's—"early onset" and "late onset." The distinction is purely chronological. A small but real percentage of Alzheimer's victims begin suffering from the illness relatively early in their lives, sometimes as early as their forties or early fifties. However, the vast majority of all cases of Alzheimer's start cropping up when patients are much older. One of the many questions puzzling scientists has been why: Why do most people who are at risk for Alzheimer's not become ill until they are in their seventies or older? Cohen and his team, using MRI scanners at McLean's Brain-Imaging Center, may have found an answer.

As in other MRI experiments with humans, the study subjects lay on their backs on a padded table with their heads inside the massive box-shaped scanner. Cohen and his colleagues were interested in the brain's use of a chemical called choline. This amino acid is essential for the normal functioning of the body's cells. It appears to be particularly important to the well-being of the neurons involved in higher cognitive functions. Obtained from our diet, choline is carried into the brain by the blood. The researchers used the MRI scanner to create one-second "snapshots" of the brain's chemical composition and neuronal activity in selected regions. They would give the subjects special choline supplements to digest and then use the MRI scanner to measure the levels of brain choline both before and after the subjects had ingested the extra choline.

They observed something quite interesting: Choline levels rose dramatically in the brains of younger adults after they ate the supplements and hardly at all in the brains of the elderly subjects. It is clear, says Cohen, that the brain's ability to metabolize or use choline declines with age. Most of us get a little bit "slower" mentally as we get older; our brains' declining ability to use choline effectively may be the culprit behind this common failing of old age. For those with Alzheimer's it could be a crucial natural shortcoming. Cohen himself thinks that this choline shortfall, uncovered with MRI technology, is a key "physical reason why people who are genetically predisposed to Alzheimer's disease are more at risk" as they get older.

RECENT ADVANCES

During the early 1990s a series of medical advances resulted in new techniques for identifying or diagnosing Alzheimer's disease. One is "burst MRI," a form of magnetic resonance imaging that takes just a few minutes and can be done with ordinary MRI scanners. PET scanning can also detect brain changes that correlate with Alzheimer's, but the process takes several hours of setup time and, as with all PET scans, uses radioisotopes. Developed by Jozef H. Duyn and his associates at the National Institutes of Health, burst MRI images the entire brain with fairly good resolution in less than two seconds and, of course, does not use radioactive compounds.

In 1995, Daniel R. Weinberger and his colleagues at the National Institutes of Mental Health reported on their use of burst MRI in a test of eight patients. Weinberger found that the technique clearly revealed lower than normal blood flow in some brain areas of people with probable Alzheimer's as compared to the brains of healthy people. Though a good first step, Weinberger notes that the technique may not be able to help in cases in which there's some doubt about an Alzheimer's diagnosis. However, if it does turn out to have a high degree of accuracy, burst MRI will be a relatively inexpensive method for detecting early brain changes caused by Alzheimer's. Most people with suspected Alzheimer's usually get an MRI scan, anyway, and burst MRI can be done with the kinds of scanners normally used in hospitals.

Using imaging technology to diagnose the illness has one overriding shortcoming. The disease must already have caused enough damage in the brain for PET or MRI to be helpful. Other researchers are using different techniques for an even earlier diagnosis of Alzheimer's. For example, a company in San Francisco called Athena Neurosciences is developing a test that detects the presence of two proteins in the cerebrospinal fluid. High levels of a protein called beta-amyloid would be a strong indication that the person does not have Alzheimer's. The presence of high levels of a protein called tau would suggest that the person does have the disease. Another test being developed by Athena would look for the presence of the apoE-4 blood protein. This test would merely provide an estimate of how likely a person is to develop Alzheimer's.

Another kind of test is being developed by researchers at Harvard Medical School, including Huntington Potter and Leonard Scinto. Their test uses tiny amounts of a chemical similar to atropine called tropicamide. Ophthalmologists and other eye specialists often use tropicamide to dilate a person's eyes during examinations. Potter and his colleagues recently found that an extremely diluted solution of tropicamide is enough to dilate the eyes of people with probable Alzheimer's. Potter had previously observed that many people with Down syndrome, a genetically caused form of mental retardation, often develop Alzheimer's symptoms as they age. People with Down syndrome are also very sensitive to chemicals that inhibit the activity of the brain neurotransmitter acetylcholine. Tropicamide is just such a compound. The high sensitivity of Alzheimer's patients to tropicamide fits well with the fact that Alzheimer's destroys neurons that produce acetylcholine. If this tests turns out to be reliable, it would be many times cheaper and easier to administer than burst MRI scans.

An even more recent advance was announced in March 1996 by researchers at the Good Samaritan Regional Medical Center in Phoenix, Arizona. Led by Eric Reiman, the team used PET to examine thirty-three people in their fifties and sixties who had no outward signs of Alzheimer's disease. Their thinking and reasoning abilities were perfectly normal. However, eleven people in the group carried two copies of the apoE-4 gene in their genetic codes. The other twenty-two had no copies of apoE-4. People carrying two copies of the apoE-4 gene are obviously the most at risk to develop Alzheimer's.

Reiman and his team knew that PET scans and MRI scans had already been used to image differences between the brains of healthy people and those with probable Alzheimer's. What he and his colleagues did was put these two pieces of the puzzle together. First, they got PET images of the brains of their thirty-three subjects. Then they used a powerful computer program to "adjust" all the PET images to the same shape, superimpose those images one on the other, and finally produce a composite PET map. This composite map revealed the brain regions that malfunction in those at risk for Alzheimer's (those people with the two copies of the apoE-4 gene).

According to Reiman, the people with the two copies of apoE-4 had unusually low levels of activity in the same parts of the brain as another group of patients already in the throes of the disease. What's more, the same group of eleven people with the two copies of apoE-4 also had changes in brain activity similar to those seen in people who are very old. Reiman speculates that the apoE-4 allele may somehow speed up certain aging processes. Thus, it appears that Alzheimer's disease is a form of superadvanced brain aging. Your body may be 65, but your brain is 105 and getting older faster by the day.

If Reiman's findings are confirmed, it may be possible to use a combination of PET scans and genetic testing to determine if a person has a high risk of developing Alzheimer's—and even tell if the unseen, rapid brain aging is already starting to take place. While this would not be helpful information today, it will be eventually. Researchers will someday, perhaps soon, develop effective treatments that can retard or even stop the brain changes caused by Alzheimer's. Then these kinds of tests will give people the chance to make the changes in diet or medication needed to finally stop this terrible scourge.

MENTAL ILLNESSES AND THE BRAIN

Alzheimer's disease affects nearly 3 million Americans directly, and many times that number of their relatives and friends suffer with them. It is a physical illness that causes detectable physical changes in the brains of the Alzheimer's patient. Just as devastating, however, are those brain breakdowns that have long been tagged as "mental" illnesses—diseases of the mind. Like Alzheimer's and other chronic so-called physical brain disorders, such as Parkinson's disease and epilepsy, mental illness disrupts the lives of many millions of Americans.

A mental illness can be defined as abnormal behavior or disturbing feelings, thoughts, or actions that interfere with a person's ability to live his or her daily life. Of course, the definition of "abnormal" depends heavily on cultural and social values. Defining "abnormal" can also be politically manipulated—and often is. The sorry history in many countries of psychiatric imprisonment of politically unpopular people is proof enough. In general, though, people who are chronically unable to handle their daily responsibilities because they suffer from disturbing or intrusive thoughts or feelings are probably exhibiting abnormal behavior no matter what the society, culture, or political fashion. Mental illness is far from uncommon. Probably between 16 and 25 percent of all Americans suffer from some form of mental illness.

Mental illness is just that—an illness. It is not demonic possession. Neither is it playacting, laziness, or some other behavior that the person controls. We now know that many mental illnesses have a genetic component; they run in families. They may also have environmental components. Simply having a gene or genes that predispose one to a mental illness does not mean one will come down with it. Some environmental "trigger" or cofactor may also be necessary to set it off. Because mental illnesses are illnesses, a specific abnormal behavior is called a symptom. A combination of several symptoms is known as a syndrome, and most mental disorders are syndromes.

The medical community recognizes more than 250 mental disorders, which are classified into different types or groups. These include:

- *Adjustment disorders*, which develop in response to a specific event, such as the death of a relative or the loss of a job;
- *Affective disorders*, such as clinical or severe depression, which have to do with disturbances of mood;
- *Anxiety disorders*, which cause a person to experience tension, fear, and feelings of danger;
- *Dissociative disorders*, including those having to do with the splitting of a person's psychological functions (such as memory or knowledge of identity) from the rest of the personality; psychogenic amnesia is an example;
- *Personality disorders*, such as antipersonal personality disorder, which are enduring problems with relating to the social environment;
- *Psychosexual disorders*, including a number of sexual dysfunctions in which psychological factors play a major role;
- *Psychotic disorders*, including those that affect a person's contact with reality; schizophrenia is the most prominent of these disorders;
- *Somatoform disorders*, involving bodily malfunctions, such as breathing difficulties or pains that have no apparent physical cause; the most common is hypochondriasis, a constant fear of disease;
- *Substance-use disorders*, including chemical dependence on, or abuse of, alcohol, drugs, or tobacco.

Among the most common mental illnesses are schizophrenia and clinical depression. They are also the most intensively studied. Recent breakthroughs in both imaging techniques and drug therapies are offering new glimmers of hope to the millions of people who suffer from these brain-based disorders.

PET AND SEVERE DEPRESSION

Everyone feels depressed at different times during their lives. But for millions of people depression is not an occasional occurrence. It lasts years, decades. This kind of depression is qualitatively different from the "bummer" moods that come and go. The feelings of apathy, hopelessness, and bleakness are like a dark curtain across daily experience. The signs and symptoms of severe or clinical depression wax and wane but never go completely away. Psychologists and others suspect that the vast majority of people who commit suicide do so in the midst of a bout of severe depression.

Several teams of genetic scientists have uncovered signs of a genetic link to clinical depression. They've been encouraged by the work of other researchers who have compiled an impressive array of evidence pointing to the essential biochemical nature of severe depression. That evidence points to a chronic disruption in the levels of the neurotransmitter chemical serotonin in the brain. A new family of medications called serotonin reuptake inhibitors have had dramatically positive effects for many thousands of people suffering from clinical depression. These drugs include Prozac and Zoloft, and they essentially prevent the reabsorption of serotonin after it has been used by certain neurons to transmit signals across the synaptic gap.

One fascinating question for neuroscientists has been exactly what parts of the brain are involved in severe depression. In 1992, Washington University's Wayne Drevets and his colleagues provided an answer using PET. Drevets worked with two groups of people on this PET investigation. The control group consisted of thirty-three people who had no history of clinical depression. The study group was made up of twenty-three adults. Thirteen were suffering from severe depression at the time of the tests. The other ten had been diagnosed with severe depression but were not suffering from any symptoms at the time. All twenty-three in the group had at least one parent, child, or brother or sister who also suffered from clinical depression. None had any family history of other psychiatric problems, and none of the people in the test group had taken any medications for their depression for at least three weeks.

The first part of Drevets's investigation focused on six people in the test group and eighteen people from the control group. Because they didn't know exactly which part of the brain to look at, the researchers did whole-brain PET scans on the subjects. A special computer program combined the different scans together, minimizing individual differences and giving the neuroscientists a composite view of the blood flow in the brains of each group. Then they compared the composites from each group.

What they found was significantly heightened blood flow in the left prefrontal cortex of all six currently depressed people from the clinical depression group but no increase in that brain area in the control group. This gave Drevets and his people a target on which to focus in the next round.

For the second part of the experiment, the researchers did PET scans on the remaining seven currently depressed people and the other fifteen controls. Once again, they saw dramatically increased blood flow in the left prefrontal cortex of the clinically depressed people, compared to the controls.

Finally, the researchers looked at PET scans of the people whose clinical depression was not active and compared those scans with those from the currently depressed subjects as well as the controls. Drevets and his group uncovered another difference. Those subjects whose depression was in remission had stable blood flow in their left prefrontal cortex. But all the people in the clinical-depression group had high activity in their amygdalas. (As we saw in chapter 9, the amydala is a part of the brain's limbic system that is Emotion Central.)

Drevets believes that the left prefrontal cortex may be processing the constant flow of negative thoughts that course through the minds of severely depressed people. An active left prefrontal cortex, he adds, is an indication that a major depressive episode is in progress. At the same time, he says, the elevated blood flow to the amygdala seen by the PET scans suggests that a person may have a genetic propensity to clinical depression. The people who suffered the most severe symptoms of clinical depression were also those with the most active amygdalas. This suggests that the amygdala somehow plays a major role in the severity of clinical depression.

THE TRAGEDY OF SCHIZOPHRENIA

My Aunt Joan suffered from schizophrenia, a word that literally means "split mind." However, she did not have multiple personalities. The name itself is misleading and dates from a time when doctors did not understand the nature of this illness. Schizophrenia is a mental illness characterized by impairments of thinking and mood in which a person's perceptions of reality and of daily events become seriously distorted. The typical symptoms include bizarre delusions, often dealing with being followed, stared at, or persecuted by authority figures; visual and aural hallucinations which last for hours or days at a time; a flattening of emotions or inappropriate emotional displays; and a continuously decreasing ability to function normally at work or in social situations. It is obvious to those who have long known them that people with schizophrenia undergo a profound change. In a real sense, they become different people.

Schizophrenia is probably the most common of all the psychotic disorders and the most difficult to treat. Though in some cases the illness doesn't begin until middle age, the symptoms usually start appearing when a person is a teenager. Psychiatrists refer to the beginning of the illness as "the psychotic break," and it can be quite dramatic. The person can go from perfectly normal to utterly psychotic in a matter of months. From then on until the end of his or her life, the person will probably never be free of the illness. Though the symptoms may wax and wane over the years, permanent remissions are extremely rare.

People with schizophrenia slide into an inner world of fantasy and delusions. They may exhibit a loosening of associations, with their conversations leaping from one unrelated idea to another. Their speech is often repetitive, abstract, or vague; they play with language, making up nonsense words. Schizophrenics frequently experience hallucinations and often hear voices which may tell them to carry out bizarre or distructive actions. Their body movements—or lack thereof—may become strange. Some people appear rigid, while others may grimace or have odd mannerisms, and rocking and pacing are common behaviors. The illness appears to be equally common in both genders.

One of the leading researchers in the field of schizophrenia and the brain is Nancy Andreasen, a professor of psychiatry and the director of the Mental Health Clinical Research Center at the University of Iowa Hospitals and Clinics. Andreasen has accurately noted that no illlness is defined by a single symptom, but rather by a unique constellation of them. But the symptoms of schizophrenia are so diverse that a hundred years ago they confounded any description of the illness. Two symptoms considered hallmarks of schizophrenia, hallucinations and delusions, have still to be clearly tied to one another by some physical cause or mechanism. Not only do the symptoms of this illness range in severity and prominence from person to person; they also affect nearly every aspect of a person's experience and daily life. Some other mental disorders, such as clinical depression or obsessive-compulsive disorder, often can be controlled with medications. People with these conditions can often go on to lead normal or nearly normal lives. Schizophrenia, though, is an illness that has resolutely resisted any effective drug treatment.

It is no surprise, then, that many brain researchers have turned their attention and their brain-imaging machines to mental illnesses. In an increasingly large number of cases they are beginning to uncover some of the biological underpinnings of some of these disorders. Schizophrenia is one of them.

SPECT AND SCHIZOPHRENIA

SPECT stands for single photon emission computed tomography. (Some scientists drop the "Computed" and refer to it as SPET.) SPECT is much less expensive than PET; it doesn't require that the hospital or medical center have a million-dollar cyclotron on hand to produce radioactive isotopes. SPECT is also a lot easier than PET to actually carry out. At the same time, many of the medical imaging tasks done with PET can also be carried out with SPECT equipment. It can help doctors diagnose and evaluate many brain disorders besides schizophrenia, including Alzheimer's disease, epilepsy, and various tumors. Some researchers are also using SPECT to learn more about the brain's growth and development.

Like PET, SPECT also detects photons, but not photons released in pairs. This imaging technique instead involves the detection of gamma rays emitted singly from radioisotopes, such as technetium 99m and thallium 201. These radioisotopes are incorporated into proteins or molecules (called radiopharmaceuticals) that certain organs normally use.

As many as three photon-sensitive cameras, commonly called gamma cameras, rotate around a patient's head, detecting the photons as they fly out of the brain. A powerful computer program calculates the information about the photons' position, angle of flight, and energy and creates a series of two-dimensional slices through the brain. The program then stacks these slices into a three-dimensional image. The image shows the distribution of the radioisotope that was injected into the patient.

IMAGING MADNESS

Not surprisingly, some researchers have started using brain-imaging techniques to study schizophrenia. The potpourri of results provides a striking look at the difficulties of this kind of scientific endeavor. Different researchers using different imaging methods seem to be getting different results. For example, some MRI scans have revealed abnormalities in certain regions of the left temporal lobes of people with schizophrenia, particularly in the hippocampus, the parahippocampal gyrus, and the superior temporal gyrus. The latter two sites are on the folds or wrinkles of neural tissue in the left temporal lobe. Other researchers have used PET and SPECT scans to try and uncover some of the functional connections between these abnormalities and schizophrenia. These images have often added to the confusing picture of the brain and schizophrenia.

In 1992, for example, several researchers produced PET images of the brains of schizophrenic patients who suffered from hallucinations. Depending on the radioactive tracers used and the techniques applied, PET can image either blood flow in a brain region or a region's metabolic rate—that is, how fast the neurons are firing. Some of these people had high levels of blood flow in the parahippocampal gyrus. These same patients had unusually low rates of blood flow in the inferior frontal cortex (a part of the frontal lobe lying beneath the surface of the brain). This abnormally low blood flow corresponded to some nonhallucinatory symptoms. Patients in another PET study turned out to have lower than normal neural activity in the hippocampus itself but normal activity in the inferior frontal lobe. In still another PET study, researchers looked at the brains of schizophrenic patients while they were experiencing auditory hallucinations. Auditory hallucinations are quite common in schizophrenia and often consist of voices telling the person to do something harmful. In this study, the researchers found unusually low brain activity in Wernicke's area in the left temporal lobe. As we saw in the chapter on language, Wernicke's area is an important brain region for speech comprehension. The same study also found an increase in brain activity in the region of the right temporal lobe that corresponds to Broca's area but nothing unusual in Broca's area itself. Like Wernicke's area, Broca's area is also an important brain region for language.

A 1993 study using SPECT scans examined the brains of people with schizophrenia as they were experiencing auditory hallucinations. The SPECT scans showed increased blood flow in the left superior temporal gyrus (one of the wrinkles of neural tissue in the left temporal lobe) while the auditory hallucinations were taking place. Blood-flow levels returned to normal after the patients took their medications. Still another 1993 SPECT study uncovered a slightly different brain-activity pattern. Three British researchers at King's College Hospital in London, led by P. K. McGuire, also used SPECT to examine schizophrenic patients while they were hearing voices. In McGuire's study, the SPECT images showed increased cerebral blood flow in Broca's area during the auditory hallucinations.

Is there any pattern to this? In fact, there is. Most of the MRI, PET and SPECT studies of people with schizophrenia reveal a strong connection between auditory hallucinations and unusual brain activity in the left temporal lobe. McGuire suggests that these findings fit well with the psychological concept called "inner speech." Essentially, inner speech is the subjective act of talking to oneself without speaking aloud. According to this concept, when we begin to think a thought, the neural impulses making up that "intended thought" first move out from the various language subsystems in the brain. The brain gives the intended thought a basic linguistic form via regions that supply information about word meanings, grammar, and vocabulary. The thought then acquires a speechlike representation from regions that store basic phonological or speech-sound information. It is at this point that the intended thought becomes inner or subvocal speech. At the same time, a kind of "feedforward loop" sends this information to other areas of the brain that recognize the thought and its associated inner speech as self-generated. In this way, I recognize that the "voice" I hear as I think thoughts is my own voice, my inner voice; myself thinking.

The same process can happen in reverse. That is, subvocal or inner speech will be captured and processed by the brain's auditory cortex and language-processing subsystems while its meaning and vocabulary is analyzed by various semantic and grammatical neural subsystems. But what if your feed-forward mechanism goes awry? Then your brain would not know that the subvocal speech was generated by the brain itself. You would not have any sense of "ownership" for the thoughts being uttered by your own inner voice. The result: auditory hallucinations, the sense that you are hearing "voices" that are not your own. Nor are these voices necessarily "inside your head." Since your brain *doesn't know* that it is the very source of the voices, they would be indistinguishable from the voices of people on the street, on the radio, or coming from the TV set.

Some PET studies of normal individuals have suggested that Broca's area plays an important role in subvocal speech. So have some MRI images of the brain. SPECT images point to a breakdown in the left temporal lobe—the location of Broca's area—as an important component of a major aspect of schizophrenia.

SCHIZOPHRENIA AND THE GATEWAY TO THE BRAIN

Nancy Andreasen believes that the many different brain-imaging techniques are providing a new picture of schizophrenia and its possible cause in the brain. "The full range of schizophrenia's symptoms *could* arise from abnormalities in brain circuitry for processing information and focusing attention," she has said. The inability to focus attention is one of the typical symptoms of schizophrenia.

Researchers in Andreasen's laboratory are exploring a new hypothesis for the cause of schizophrenia. It's supported by four large studies using MRI, two of which were completed in 1994; recent PET studies; and the findings of several other researchers. Andreasen's hypothesis is that schizophrenia's symptoms arise from misconnections in some of the brain's circuitry. The brain structures Andreasen thinks are involved include the corpus callosum and the thalamus. The corpus callosum is the main cable of nerve tissue that connects the brain's two cerebral hemispheres. The thalamus, as we've already found, is what Andreasen calls "the gateway to the brain," for it monitors nearly all incoming sensory information, which it then sends on to the proper brain regions.

Andreasen and other researchers have found that, compared with healthy volunteers, schizophrenics have abnormalities in these and other so-called midline structures. A very common one is enlargement of the brain's ventricles, the cavities deep within the brain's center that contain cerebrospinal fluid. During the brain's formation, nerve cells originate and migrate outward from these ventricles. An early 1986 study with MRI by Andreasen and her colleagues was one of the first to suggest that schizophrenia was, at its root, a developmental disorder of the brain rather than some kind of degenerative disease, like Alzheimer's, that involved the death of neurons. Other CT scan and MRI studies later added weight to this suggestion.

Andreasen and her colleagues have been busy exploring this hypothesis in considerable depth, using recent advances in MRI and some new computer software. They have been able to combine different brain images to produce what she has called "three-dimensional, detailed composites of 'an average schizophrenic brain' and an 'average normal brain.' " As they expected, they found more cerebrospinal fluid and less total brain tissue in the average schizophrenic brain than in the average normal brain. But this finding raised another question: Do the enlarged ventricles represent loss of brain tissue in general— or in the surrounding midline structures—due to some injury or developmental defect?

The answer came from the brain images. "The most striking [midline-structure anomaly] is a partial or complete lack of development in the corpus callosum," Andreasen has said. "Such a severe disruption in circuitry between the brain's hemispheres may explain why some schizophrenics respond poorly to medications." Another abnormality found by both Andreasen and other researchers is a smaller-than-normal thalamus in the brains of schizophrenics. She has noted that the thalamus is crucial to relaying information and is linked to the prefrontal cortex, which in turn is involved in the integration of thoughts.

An inability to categorize incoming information according to its importance or to filter out irrelevant information could account for a person's inability to properly focus attention. In other words, you must have some idea of what's important and what's not if you want to keep the wheat and ignore the chaff. Other research has also implicated "attention circuitry" in the brain, specifically neurons in the brain stem that control posture and the regions which regulate emotional responsiveness.

In 1995, Andreasen and her colleagues decided to look at what happens in the brain when a person tries to focus his or her attention. This study was very similar to the ones reported in chapter 6 that looked at the sensory phenomenon of perfect pitch. If a person has a different sound piped into each ear, he or she will normally report hearing the sound presented in the right ear. Andreasen and her team took PET scans of people who were asked to listen for words or meaningless syllables with their *left* ear. What she found was "marked shifts in patterns of activity for speech-processing areas in the normal listeners but no similar shift in the patients with schizophrenia."

Like any good scientist, Andreasen has been cautious about conclusions. Her "attention dysfunction" hypothesis is a preliminary one, she has said. But it is consistent with the PET and MRI images that implicate the thalamus and the corpus callosum "attention circuits" in schizophrenia. Disruptions in the normal functioning of these areas of the brain, she feels, could very well lead to hallucinations, delusions, disorganization of speech and behavior, and what are called "negative symptoms"—capacities a person normally has that are lessened in schizophrenia, such as the capacity for enjoying life.

If Andreasen's hypothesis is correct, schizophrenia is more than just a breakdown in the brain's normal functioning. That such breakdowns are taking place is incontrovertible. MRI, SPECT, and PET scans all reveal abnormal activity in several brain regions. They include the left temporal lobe, which plays such a crucial role in language and processing speech sounds; the prefrontal lobe, which integrates the various aspects of what we call conscious thought; and "attention circuits," which include the brain stem, the limbic system (the cingulate gyrus and the thalamus), and the corpus callosum.

More than all this, though, is the intriguing evidence that some of these attention circuits never developed normally in the first place. Does the well-known "psychotic break" in schizophrenia take place in adolescence because the underdeveloped corpus callosum can no longer handle the flood of data flowing between the two cerebral hemispheres? Do visual and auditory hallucinations occur because the smaller-than-normal thalamus does a poor job as the brain's sensory gateway? Do schizophrenics lack the ability to focus their attention on the tasks at hand in their daily lives because their brain's attentional circuits cannot identify what tasks are the important ones?

My Aunt Joan lived all her adult life trapped in the prison of her mind, unable to ever free herself from the symptoms of schizophrenia. Her parents, my father and his sister, and to a lesser degree her nieces and nephews all suffered with her. The work being done by

Nancy Andreasen, P. K. McGuire, and others came far too late to help her.

But in the months and years to come, researchers like McGuire and Andreasen will use the new brain-imaging technologies to answer some of these questions. From those answers will eventually come new medications and more effective treatments for this mental disorder that afflicted Joan Davis and still plagues more than 2 million Americans.

CHAPTER 12

THE TERRITORY OF THE MIND

NEUROSCIENTISTS have known for decades that certain brain diseases or injuries can profoundly change an individual's personality. People who suffer from Alzheimer's disease slowly but inexorably lose their *selves*. The person we used to know eventually disappears. The personality disintegrates. The mind goes. People suffering from mental illnesses such as schizophrenia also undergo profound changes in their personalities. In these cases, also, the people we once knew effectively disappear, so profound are the changes to their minds.

But before medical science gained an understanding of Alzheimer's or began traveling the long road to an enlightened understanding of schizophrenia, there was a man named Phineas Gage. The horrendous injury he suffered, and its tragic consequences, proved to be a watershed in our understanding of the connection between the brain and the mind.

THE TAMPING ROD

Phineas Gage was a young man who worked for the Rutland and Burlington Railroad in New England. One day in September 1848, Gage was setting up a dynamite charge as part of his job. As he tamped down the blasting powder into the hole with an inch-thick iron rod, he accidentally tamped it a little too hard. The powder exploded and flung the rod back up into his face. And *through* his face. The metal rod smashed through his left cheek, took out his left eye, and flew out the top of his skull. Gage fell to the ground—and moments later got up again. His fellow workers rushed him into the nearby town, where a doctor named John Harlow treated the man's wounds as best he could. Harlow was stunned by the sight. He could put the index fingers of each hand into the holes in Gage's face and head and touch his fingertips together inside the man's skull. Yet the man sat there in front of him, alive and talking.

Phineas Gage survived his horrific injury, but not as Phineas Gage. True, he retained all the intelligence and memories of his preaccident life. He had no problems with body movements or any other physical functions. His language ability was completely normal, and his sensory perceptions (with the exception of vision; he had lost an eye, after all) seemed unaffected. But the gentle, friendly man, God-fearing and responsible, was gone. The "new" Phineas Gage was a loudmouthed liar, completely irresponsible and given to boasting and profanity. He quickly lost his job on the Rutland and Burlington and never held another. For the next dozen years he wandered across the country, cadging meals and money where he could, living the life of a bum—in contemporary terms, a homeless person. He never recovered from his injury, nor did the "old" Phineas Gage ever "return" to occupy his body.

Gage died in 1861 from the effects of an epileptic seizure. Several years later, John Harlow heard about the death of his patient and persuaded Gage's family to exhume the remains. Gage's brain was long gone, but his skull remained. The family donated it for medical research. Harlow was convinced that the changes in Gage's personality had been caused by damage to his frontal lobes. But his was a minority opinion in the 1860s. Some of his detractors doubted that the injury to Phineas Gage had even occurred.

For more than a century Gage's skull and the infamous tamping rod remained in the Warren Medical Museum at Harvard University. The story of Phineas Gage became a classic in neurology textbooks. His injury and its consequences inspired generations of medical researchers to probe more deeply the neurological underpinnings of the human personality and the human mind.

But no one really knew *exactly* what happened to cause the dramatic changes in Phineas Gage. In 1994, 146 years after Gage was speared by the tamping rod, Antonio and Hanna Damasio decided that they might be able to answer that question. Hanna Damasio, the computer expert of the husband-and-wife team, created a detailed computer model of Phineas Gage's skull. She also used computer software to simulate the paths that the tamping rod could have taken as it passed through the skull and the brain.

The rod could have taken several paths, the Damasios found. The most likely one, though, would have missed the areas in the left frontal and temporal lobes responsible for language and some motor skills. However, it appears that the rod passed right through and devastated a portion of the left prefrontal area of the brain, lying in front of the left sensorimotor cortex and Broca's area. It would have also seriously damaged the left orbitofrontal cortex, a part of the underside of the left frontal lobe.

The Damasios had already seen damage to similar areas of the brain in a dozen of their own patients, damage caused by strokes, illnesses, and accidents of various kinds (though none from tamping rods). The pattern of mental and personality changes were the same as those that happened to Phineas Gage more than a century ago. The patients retained normal intellectual function, language skills, and motor abilities, but their personalities changed drastically. They became loud, abusive, asocial, and irresponsible.

"Gage's story was the historical beginnings of the study of the biological basis of behavior," Antonio Damasio was quoted as saying in an article in *Discover* magazine, "and the location of his lesion had always been a mystery." Now that mystery has been solved.

But not completely. S. Clifford Schold Jr. is the chairman of the Department of Neurology at the University of Texas Southwestern Medical Center at Dallas. "Although we now recognize the neurological syndrome exhibited by Gage," Schold recently wrote in a World Wide Web publication, "we have still not succeeded in developing a comprehensive concept of the function of this area of the brain.

"Exactly what is this 'silent area' of the brain doing in those of us who have not had Phineas's misfortune?" Schold asks. ("Silent" is a euphemism for "we don't understand its function.") "What does it mean to act 'appropriately' in a social setting? Can we develop an operational definition of 'judgment'? Do anatomic, biochemical, or physiological variations in this [brain] area account for the range of social behavior we encounter every day?"

Concludes Schold: "The ghost of the brain of Phineas Gage means two things to me: The frontal lobes remain a great mystery, and one well-studied and considered patient can produce enormous insights in human medicine."

THE MIND: DUALISM OR MATERIALISM?

The tragedy of Phineas Gage nearly 150 years ago and the brain injuries and breakdowns that affect millions of people today offer neuroscientists a compelling argument for an intimate relationship between the mind and the brain. That relationship, most researchers believe, is not mystical but materialistic. The mind is a product of the brain's activity; or perhaps it *is* the brain's activity. It is not, most brain scientists are convinced, some nonmaterial entity that has some kind of existence independent of the brain.

This contemporary scientific paradigm for the mind is one that many nonscientists have difficulty both understanding and accepting. How can the mind *not* be something separate from the body or the brain? It certainly *feels* real to us. We know we have free will, that with our minds we can make decisions and choices that are not irrevocably governed by our bodies or outside influences. We *are* the masters of our fates, are we not, and the captains of our souls? While often it may not seem that way, most of us most of the time are convinced by our own inner and subjective experiences that this is true.

At the same time, millions of Americans and untold billions of other humans believe in the existence of some sort of afterlife. In particular, most Christians and Muslims believe that the human personality itself survives death. For this to be true in any sense, then the mind must somehow survive beyond death, for the mind is certainly an integral part of the human personality.

That is a real sticking point for most brain researchers and other scientists. For all the evidence clearly points to the mind being something integral to the brain and its functioning; and those functions no more survive beyond the brain's death than the flame exists after the campfire burns out. The mind, for most scientists, is a term that stands for the totality of a person's conscious and unconscious mental states. This is the nondualist or materialist theory of the mind. The mind and the body are one; the mind is a product of the brain.

The philosophical theory known as dualism holds that two kinds of "substance" exist: physical objects and minds. Physical objects are material and exist in space and time. Minds are nonmaterial or spiritual. A person consists of these two substances, mind and physical object or body, but it's the mind that is essential to a person. The mind is the repository of the personality. If a person's body dies, the mind can continue to exist, but if the mind ceases to exist, then the person does, too. Bodies can exist without minds, says the dualist. And minds can exist without bodies.

Dualism has a long history in Western philosophical thought. It has been in and out of vogue many times over the centuries. The Greek philosopher Anaxagoras was the first Western thinker to distinguish between the mind and body. The most influential arguments for the dualism of mind and body come from the writings of Plato. This great Greek philosopher offered several arguments for his version of dualism. In the *Phaedo*, for example, Plato has Socrates offering the "cyclical argument." Living has an opposite: being dead. By applying the general principle that opposites arise from each other, Socrates argues that "living people are born from the dead no less than dead people from the living." This is evidence for the existence of reincarnation, which in turn implies mind-body dualism. A similar argument in the *Phaedo* is his "argument from opposites." Socrates, Plato's spokesman, asks his companion Cebes what it is that makes a living body alive. Cebes replies that it's the soul. Plato's version of dualism essentially equates the mind with the soul. If the soul gives rise to life, Socrates responds, then the soul cannot itself die—any more than an even number can also be an odd number. Thus, says Socrates, the soul must be immortal.

In both the *Phaedo* and the *Meno*, Plato presents the "recollection argument." Essentially, says Plato through the person of Socrates, we can know the correct answers to some questions when we haven't been taught the answers beforehand. This is evidence that all knowledge is a form of recollection, the remembering of information we learned in some nonphysical world. This, in turn, argues for the immortality of the soul and the reality of reincarnation.

Plato's mind-body idea fits well with his theory of Forms. Plato argued that ordinary physical objects are actually examples or "shadows" of perfect ideas he called Forms. The world of our senses is thus less real than this ideal reality of Forms. Before our birth, Plato said, our souls were in constant and immediate contact with these perfect Forms. When we are born and our souls enter our bodies, they lose that immediate connection and are plunged into ignorance. When we die, our souls regain their connection with the Forms.

Dualism in the modern philosophical and scientific sense has its roots in the thoughts and writings of the seventeenth-century philosopher and mathematician René Descartes. Disgusted with the then current state of what passed for science, Descartes became determined to discover some kind of "first principle," a basic statement of truth that could not be doubted. On this first principle, he thought, humanity would be able to build a body of indisputable knowledge. He finally found one statement that he himself could not doubt: "I think, therefore I am." This statement became the basis of his philosophical and mathematical work, and that work eventually shaped the world we live in today.

When Descartes concluded that "I think, therefore I am," he provided himself with a starting point for all his subsequent mathematical and philosophical positions. He proceeded, using his method of scientific deduction, to build a philosophical system consisting of two distinct orders of reality. God and the human mind belonged to one order of reality; nature belonged to the other. Nature, Descartes felt, was a mechanism that mathematics could explain. However, some entities could not be explained by mathematics. God was one; the mind was another. Thus, said Descartes (a deeply spiritual man), these spiritual entities belonged to another type of reality. Moreover, the mind—this separate reality—can and does exert influence over matter; namely, the brain and the body.

It is this position, that mind and matter are separate realities and that the mind can control the brain and body, that most neuroscientists cannot accept. And the reason, to their minds, is simple. The evidence they see does not support such a position. It supports a more materialistic one: that mind is an emergent property of a particular piece of matter, the piece called the brain.

This opposition to dualism is not new in science. The current materialist paradigm of the mind goes back to at least the eighteenth century. In 1749 the French philosopher Denis Diderot described his materialist philosophy in his *Letter on the Blind*. (That same year, the British scientist David Hartley first used the word "psychology" in its modern sense in his book *Observations on Man*.) In 1758 the French philosopher Claude-Adrien Helvétius wrote *Essays on the Mind*, in which he endorsed the idea that the mind develops as a result of the sensations it perceives rather than because of any innate tendencies. The English Parliament condemned the book, and it was publicly burned in France.

The Scottish philosopher, historian, and economist James Mill published *Analysis of the Phenomena of the Human Mind* in 1829. In this book Mill tried to prove that the mind was no more than a machine, without any creative function. Eleven years later, the German physiologist Johannes Peter Müller offered a mechanistic explanation of human thinking in his *Handbook of Human Psychology*. And in 1899 Ernest Haeckel, the famous German biologist, declared, in *The Riddle of the Universe*, that the mind is a product of the body and does not survive the body's death.

THEORIES OF THE MIND

Brain researchers have always had some interest in the nature of the mind; it goes with the territory. The same is true of philosophers and philosophy, but in spades; philosophy's been at the mind game for many centuries. The recent revolution in our biological and neurological understanding of the brain has served to bring these two sometimes disparate fields somewhat closer together. The common ground has been the nature of the mind.

So many theories of the mind are afoot today that an entire book could be written about them. In fact, several have, though this is not one of them. However, it's worth our while to take a quick look at some of the more popular, curious, or downright strange theories of the mind that are currently in vogue.

The theorists who offer these proposals fit into two main categories: the materialists and the mysterians. The materialists essentially hold that the mind is a product of the brain. Because the mind is a physical, material process, it is at least theoretically possible for science to eventually understand its nature. The mysterians (the name was given to them by philosopher Owen Flanagan of Duke University, after the 1960s rock group "? and the Mysterians") believe that conventional neuroscience will never be able to completely explain the nature of consciousness and the mind.

Two of the more prominent theories offered by the materialists are:

- *The Astonishing Hypothesis.* This book title is also the position taken by Nobelist Francis Crick (of DNA fame) and his colleague the German neuroscientist Christof Koch. Crick and Koch believe that consciousness and the mind arise from a combination of short-term memory and attention; this combination is the product of processes in the brain that coordinate the signaling of different neural circuits.

• *Neural Darwinism.* This is the name that neuroscientist Gerald Edelman gives to his theory of the mind. Edelman contends that awareness arises from the competition among clusters of neurons to provide an accurate model of the outside world.

The mysterians are a diverse group that includes relatively few neuroscientists (not surprisingly) and a larger number of physicists and philosophers. Among the theories offered by mysterians are:

• *Quantum consciousness.* Physicist Roger Penrose has suggested that the mind is a product of interactions taking place at the subatomic or quantum level of reality. The mind, says Penrose, can therefore never be completely understood because the nondeterministic effects of quantum actions prevent such knowledge from being attained. Most neuroscientists dismiss Penrose's theory, but it is gaining popularity among the general public.
• *"The antimaterialists."* This is as good a handle as any for the position advocated by such philosophers as Jerry Fodor of Rutgers University. Fodor argues that the mind, and our subjective experiences of the world, may never be completely explainable by *any* materialist theory, classical or quantum.
• *"The Haldane Hypothesis."* The British biologist J. B. S. Haldane once wrote that "the universe is not only queerer than we imagine; it is queerer than we *can* imagine." This aphorism aptly sums up the most extreme of the mysterian positions as advocated by philosopher Colin McGinn of Rutgers University. McGinn notes that our brains are the products of evolutionary processes. Like the brains of every other animal, ours must have certain cognitive limitations. Rats can never conceive of relativity; perhaps our minds, he says, are innately unable to understand other aspects of reality. Consciousness, the relationship between mind and matter, may be one concept we will never understand.

KAREN ANN'S LEGACY

By the time Hounsfield and Cormack had invented the CT scanner in 1973, dualism was pretty much dead as a viable paradigm for the mind-brain conundrum. Materialist theories were ascendant. Three not-so-small questions remained unanswered: *Where* in the brain does mind/consciousness/awareness originate? *How* does the mind come into existence in the brain? And *why*?

One clue to an answer to the questions where and how come from a personal tragedy that garnered global attention. On April 18, 1975, a young woman named Karen Ann Quinlan was at a party with some friends. She was drinking gin and tonics but had earlier that day taken some Valium and the painkiller drug Darvon. The combination of drugs and alcohol didn't kill her; the results were far worse than that.

In the middle of the gathering Quinlan suddenly collapsed. Her heart stopped, and her breathing ceased. By the time paramedics arrived and revived her, too much damage had already been done. Starved of oxygen for almost an hour, her brain had been permanently damaged. Quinlan had slipped into the state of profound unconsciousness called a coma. The doctors told her parents that Karen Ann would never recover consciousness. Joseph and Julia Quinlan realized that the person who had been their daughter was gone and would never return. They asked the doctors to turn off the ventilator that was helping Karen Ann breathe so she could die a natural death. Fearing a possible malpractice suit, the doctors refused. The Quinlans petitioned a New Jersey court to order the doctors to abide by their wishes. The courts finally did so, and in 1976 the ventilator was turned off.

And Karen Ann Quinlan continued breathing. By this time she had entered a level of unconsciousness doctors call a "persistent vegetative state." Her heart continued beating; her lungs continued breathing. Her body went through normal waking and sleeping cycles, and when she was "awake," her eyes would open. But Quinlan was not aware of her surroundings. Her conscious mind never returned. In 1985, ten years after her collapse, she died of massive infections.

The doctor who performed the autopsy, Robert Goode, removed Quinlan's brain and preserved it in a standard fixative called formalin. Three years later, Goode asked Hannah Kinney if she would like to study Quinlan's preserved brain. Kinney was a pathologist at Children's Hospital in Boston and had done research on the brain stem. Kinney was intrigued with the challenge. She knew that other people who had slipped into persistent vegetative states had suffered considerable damage to their cerebral cortex. Kinney hoped that by studying Quinlan's brain she could finally determine exactly what had happened in the young woman's brain thirteen years earlier. In truth, she figured that Quinlan's case would probably turn out to be the same as most others.

Kinney was wrong. When she examined sections of Quinlan's cerebral cortex under the microscope, it turned out to be pretty much undamaged. Kinney realized that whatever damage had sent Quinlan into a persistent vegetative state, it was somewhere else. She prepared the brain for more extensive study by embedding it in paraffin—the same waxy substance that people use in home canning. Then Kinney sliced Quinlan's entire brain into a set of very thin sections and mounted them on slides.

She now turned to a combination of old and new medical technology to study the brain slices, using a microscope connected to a computer. The computer ran a program that Kinney used to outline specific areas of brain tissue that she then studied through the microscope, looking for any signs of scarring or other neurological damage. She used the microscope-computer combination to create a three-dimensional map of all the locations in Quinlan's brain that contained signs of injuries. With this map, Kinney made a surprising discovery, one that sheds new light on the nature of the human mind and consciousness.

To understand what Kinney found, imagine that I have gone out to my garage to talk with the carpenter who is sanding down some kitchen cabinet doors. I step outside to talk with Oscar and look at him as we talk. The image of his face hits my eyes' retinas, and the neural impulses then travel through the optic nerves and first arrive at my thalamus. From there the impulses travel to my primary visual cortex for initial visual processing of shape, color, edges, shadows, and the other visual characteristics that comprise Oscar's unique face.

But if I am to actually recognize Oscar as Oscar, a particular part of the thalamus needs to function properly. It's called the pulvinar region. Some researchers believe that this cluster of neurons in the thalamus helps pull together all the different fragments of information arriving from the senses. It acts like one of Antonio Damasio's convergence zones or as a coordinator of information. The pulvinar region works with other parts of the cerebral cortex to combine shape, size, color, texture, and other characteristics into the coherent image that is Oscar's face.

The most significant damage that Hannah Kinney found in Karen Ann Quinlan's brain was not in the cerebral cortex. It was in the thalamus. As we saw earlier, the thalamus consists of two ovoid-shaped structures buried deep in the cerebrum. They're part of the brain's limbic system and act as a primary switching system for nearly every sensory input the brain receives. Except for smell signals, all neuronal data from all the senses first passes through the thalamus on the way to other processing regions in the brain.

Several parts of Quinlan's thalamus were severely damaged. It was, Kinney has said, as if someone had taken a laser beam and burned out just those particular areas, leaving the rest of Quinlan's brain relatively undamaged. Both the thalamus's relaying neurons and the pulvinar region were wiped out. The result was that Karen Ann Quinlan's brain was cut off from the outer world. Almost all the sensory data that first arrived at her thalamus never made it out to the rest of the brain. The regions of her cerebral cortex that processed sensory data—the visual cortex, the auditory cortex, the somatosensory cortex—never saw that information. She had slipped into a netherworld from which she could never return. Unlike some stroke patients, who recover functions because undamaged parts of their brains take over, Quinlan's brain had no "backups" for those critical parts of the thalamus.

Hannah Kinney did her work without position-emission tomography (PET), magnetic resonance imaging (MRI), the electroencephalogram (EEG), or the other brain-imaging technologies in vogue today. She used an old-fashioned medical tool, a microscope, combined with a computer and good software. But her findings about Karen Ann Quinlan's brain throw a new light on the puzzle of consciousness and mind. It is clear that the thalamus is more than just a switching yard for sensory data. It must play an important role with regions of the cerebral cortex in creating human awareness.

LANGUAGE AND CONSCIOUSNESS

In chapter 10 we explored Antonio Damasio's "convergence zone" theory of how the brain creates language. As we saw, Damasio proposes that the brain contains tiny clusters of neurons that store the instructions for combining the different parts of language into coherent speech. Different convergence zones have the instructions for combining each different speech sound or phoneme into a word, such as the three phonemes that make up the word "cup." Other convergence zones store the codes for the different rules of grammar that govern how we put words together to form understandable sentences.

The convergence-zone model is an exquisite explanation for how our brain creates and uses language. However, Damasio thinks that his theory has more to offer. He suggests that a deep connection exists between our ability to create and use language and our conscious awareness of the world around us.

A multiplicity of definitions for "consciousness" exists today. An essential feature of most of them is awareness, either of the external world and its objects or of abstract concepts (like "consciousness"). Like many of his colleagues, Antonio Damasio has pondered the nature of consciousness and its connection to the brain. He believes that consciousness has to do with what he has called the act of *attending to* a set of *coactivated sequences*. A certain pattern of neural activity represents or models some perceived experience: an object we see, a sound we hear, or a complex memory involving the smell of strawberry-rhubarb pie on a windy autumn school-day afternoon. It is one of a myriad of such neural patterns that are constantly playing themselves out in the brain. This one, though, is enhanced. It stands out against the brain's ongoing background activity like the wail of an ambulance's siren cutting through the night. We are *attending to* that siren, to that sequence of neural impulses.

Most of the time we don't attend to our daily experiences any more than we constantly pay attention to our actions as we drive the car down to the grocery store. Those events, those actions, do not stand out from the brain's background activity. They are common, repetitive, standard, not new. Some unusual event, however, *will* stand out: the car that runs the red light in front of us, the child that suddenly dashes into the street after her dog, the sudden honk of a car horn behind us. Then, says Damasio, we become *conscious*.

Language is not a necessary requirement for the mere existence of consciousness, says Damasio. Basic or rudimentary forms of consciousness can exist without it. "I'm convinced that some animals have consciousness," Damasio says. "However, they do not have consciousness at the same level that humans do. Language plays a role in the level or sophistication of consciousness." The reason, says Damasio, is that language provides a level of "distancing" between the person and the object being observed. Language "distances" the self from objects in the external world and concepts manufactured and stored in the brain. What's more, Damasio asserts that "language creates the *I* of that sense of self."

If Damasio's theory is correct, then it's fair to say that all living beings—from the paramecium to the porcupine—have some kind of consciousness. For all creatures must "attend to" novel stimuli when they occur. Moreover, all living creatures must possess at least a rudimentary sense of "self." For what is the self but that which is not "every-thing else out there"? A creature's immune system defends it from attack by either external or internal enemies, whether germs, viruses, or environmental toxins. The immune system works because the body can distinguish between self and nonself. This rudimentary self is nonverbal. Language, says Damasio, changes that.

And if this is correct, then each of us creates our *I*, our self, as we learn our mother tongue.

THE CONNECTION PRINCIPLE

Until recently, Antonio Damasio's attention to the nature of conscious-ness was somewhat unusual in neuroscience. Most cognitive researchers have tended to avoid the subject as essentially, well, subjective. John Searle does not approve of such avoidance behavior; in fact, he thinks that asking hard questions about consciousness is a very important task for neuroscientists.

Searle is a professor of philosophy at the University of California at Berkeley. He is not a popular person with many brain researchers and cognitive scientists. He is especially unpopular with the coterie of sci-entists who are advocates of "strong AI." Strong AI (which stands for artificial intelligence) is the position that the human mind is like com-puter software running in the hardware called the brain. Ergo, build the right software and the computer will be intelligent.

Searle attacks the current edifice of cognitive science, and its para-digm for the mind, for what he feels is the neglect of an essential aspect of mind: consciousness, or conscious experience. Brain researchers and cognitive scientists would much rather discuss aspects of the mind that can at least theoretically be studied in some objective fashion. Searle, on the other hand, thinks that conscious awareness may be the key to understanding the nature of the mind and its relationship to the brain.

The current paradigm, at least for the majority of people in cogni-tive science, is that the mind is a collection of specific modules or facul-ties that contain the unconscious rules for language, perception, feeling, emotions, logic, and other aspects of thought. Other unconscious aspects of the brain, such as memories, usually influence behavior and thought in somewhat clandestine fashion. Consciousness, in this view, is the ability to describe or pay attention to the unconscious rules that gov-ern the mind.

However, Searle rejects this paradigm of the mind. In its stead he offers a theory he calls the Connection Principle. The mind, or mental life, he asserts, consists of conscious states and those physiological processes that generate conscious states. Even brain states that do not usually rise to consciousness are capable of doing so. For example, the hypothalamus is mainly responsible for triggering our sensation of thirst. The nonconscious workings of the hypothalamus, however, have the ability to generate a conscious awareness: "I'm thirsty." Other nonconscious processes in the brain are totally separated from conscious awareness. The activity of neurotransmitters as they carry signals across the synaptic gap between neurons do not meet Searle's criteria for "mental" activity. They have no "intentions," as he would say, while there is some kind of intention connected with the need for assuaging thirst.

Each of us experiences the world from a unique vantage point. We see the world through our eyes, hear the world through our ears, smell and taste and touch the world through our other senses. No one else occupies our body. No one else occupies the space and time that we occupy. So consciousness is singular and essentially subjective. At the same time, Searle believes, the mind is a common feature of all human brains. Just as wetness is an essential feature of water or hardness an inherent feature of a diamond, the mind is a common feature of the brain.

Despite Searle's deep distrust of "mind like computer" analogies, one essential aspect of consciousness is like a computer. Consciousness, in Searle's model, is like an on-off logic unit. It either exists or it does not. Its value equals either 1 or 0. But that's about as far as one dares push the analogy. Once the switch is on, consciousness can exist in a variety of states. Dreams, says Searle, are one form of consciousness. "Peripheral consciousness" is another. When I am busy mowing the lawn, for example, I pay close attention to where I'm going and where my feet are in relation to the mower. Meanwhile, "a part of my mind" remains aware of the birds chirping, the feel of the breeze blowing across my shirt, my shirt on my back, and the fragments of thoughts that flit through my mind.

"Repressed consciousness" is what Searle calls the unconscious desires and conflicts that sometimes break through into our conscious experience. Most of the time they remain hidden or influence our actions and thoughts in disguised ways. The same is true of the anxieties, worries, memories, and beliefs that influence our lives. Most of the time they remain "repressed" or hidden but have the potential of rising fully into consciousness. They, too, obey Searle's Connection Principle.

The "unconscious" mental state of psychology is not some state that exists *in toto* in the brain or mind, according to Searle. It is not some kind of "virtual space" containing a storehouse of thoughts which in some fashion pop up into the "reality" of consciousness. Rather, the unconscious is the brain state made up of all the various biological and neurological processes that generate conscious experience. In other words, the brain creates consciousness instant by instant, from one moment to the next.

Searle's Connection Principle rejects the notion that the brain has sets of unconscious or nonconscious "rules" that govern certain types of perception or mental functions. One notorious example—for Searle—is Noam Chomsky's concept of a "universal grammar" underlying all languages. Chomsky is the world-famous linguist at the Massachusetts Institute of Technology, and his universal grammar° concept has revolutionized the science of linguistics. Furthermore, many recent brain breakthroughs made possible by the new imaging technologies clearly support Chomsky's basic idea: The brain contains an innate set of grammatical rules that govern the creation and generation of human languages. But these rules are not available to the conscious mind.

This is the notion that Searle rejects. For him, the idea of a universal linguistic grammar encoded in the brain is as ludicrous as the idea of a "universal visual grammar." The brain does not contain a set of unconscious rules that say, "If the object is red, you can see it, but if it's ultraviolet you cannot." In fact, some animals *do* see wavelengths of light that we humans do not. The reason we don't see ultraviolet or infrared light, says Searle, simply has to do with the inherent physical limitations of the brain and the eyes. In the same way, it is obvious that the brain is inherently able to generate language. This is a biological capacity that is encoded into the brain's structure and its neurons. But it is the brain itself and its structure that makes language possible. That same structure also limits the types of languages we can learn. There is no set of unconscious rules, Searle would argue, buried deep in our brains that says, "Oh, sorry. You're fifteen years old now, and so you are too old to learn any new language very easily." Rather, it is a function of the brain's growth, structure, and organization that makes it more and more difficult to learn a new language as we get older.

°"Grammar" as used here does not mean the tedious rules we learned in grade school. Rather, it is a technical term used in linguistics that refers to the basic rules that govern the structure of sentences.

Not surprisingly, Noam Chomsky rejects Searle's arguments against universal grammars. Even more telling, though, are the objections of some psychologists. Searle's assertion that unconscious mental states possess some kind of "intention" or "goal" which gives them the potential to become conscious appears to be just plain wrong. One example of this is the phenomenon of implicit memory. A multiple-choice test or a recall test that contains words from a previously used list can call up conscious memories in people taking such tests. Sometimes, though, the volunteers will later use the same words on other tests that don't ask for those words. An example would be a test consisting of word fragments that can be completed in various ways. The word fragment "lan-" could be completed as "lance," "land," "langour," "lanolin," "lantern," or "lanthanum" (the element with atomic number 57). If the word "lantern" appeared in an earlier test, a volunteer might unintentionally use it to finish the word fragment in the later test. However, such implicit memories do not arise because of any Searlean unconscious "intention."

CHAOS AND THE MIND

An even more provocative response to John Searle's Connection Principle of the mind and consciousness comes from two other people at the University of California at Berkeley, physiologists Walter Freeman and Christine Skarda. Freeman and Skarda think Searle's contention that the neurophysiological processes in the brain create mental states is wrong. The neurophysiological process of the brain, they contend, *are* mental states. To support their contention, Freeman and Skarda turn to one of the hottest fields in science today: chaos theory.

Chaos, in this sense, is not randomness or meaninglessness. Rather, chaos in scientific terminology is a specific mathematical state of *apparent* randomness. Buried in chaotic states, however, are the seeds of order and stability. Chaos appears to be a fundamental property of the cosmos. Nineteenth-century astronomers were convinced that, given enough information, they could plot the movements of all the planets, comets, and stars in the universe into the indefinite future. Today, though, we know that's impossible. We are inherently unable to calculate all the possible variations in the movement of a single comet that would be caused by its gravitational interactions with all the other objects in the solar system. This limits how far into the future we can plot the comet's orbit. The same inherent uncertainty applies to the more mundane realm of the weather. Small and undetectable influences on the movements of air masses in one part of the earth can have an enormous impact on the weather in another part of the planet. It's called the "butterfly effect" because theoretically a butterfly flapping its wings in Beijing will influence the weather in Los Angeles. No amount of computer power, therefore, will ever enable forecasters to accurately predict the weather more than a week or so in advance.

Recently, brain scientists have recognized that the underlying or background electrical activity in the brain is essentially chaotic in nature. This means that a very flexible energy state constantly exists within a living human brain, generated by the continuous electrochemical activity of 100 billion neurons. Freeman and Skarda suggest that the brain uses this energy state to instantly organize the activity of billions of neurons in response to different stimuli from the outside world. They have already detected this kind of chaotic electrical activity in the visual and olfactory (smell) cortexes of rabbits. In other words, this chaotic, seemingly disorganized background electrical activity spontaneously organizes itself in response to sensory input. As the brain acquires new information and new experiences and stores them in the patterns of neural activity called memories, the different patterns of chaotic electrical activity incorporates them with previous memories and thoughts to create what we call consciousness, or the mind. Thus, say Freeman and Skarda, the brain "grows" the mind out of its moment-to-moment physiological and electrical activities. The essentially chaotic nature of the brain's energy state also means that its future patterns cannot be predicted with any accuracy. The reason, say Freeman and Skarda, is the butterfly effect. The tiniest change in the brain's electrochemical balance can have profound and inherently unpredictable effects for the entire neural system. So, says Freeman, if I see Oscar's familiar face, the firing pattern of many different neural networks in my brain suddenly shifts. That shift is a change in my awareness. I *attend to* Oscar's face; it stands out from the background. I am aware of him.

Memories, thoughts, and plans; repressed consciousness and peripheral consciousness—all are products of chaotic interactions within the brain. All are real, and all are utterly immaterial. We are literally, as Shakespeare said, the stuff that dreams are made of.

HIGH-FIDELITY MODELS

"We've created EEG machines with a resolution good enough to make them useful in trying to see how major areas of the cortex communicate with each other during thought." Alan Gevins has spent most of our interview time talking about his EEG research on the operations of the brain. Now, though, he is turning to the topic of the mind. It is one that is close to his heart.

"For example," he continues, "I'd like to know how the left superior parietal cortex is talking with the left dorsolateral prefrontal cortex, which is talking with the right parietal cortex. Why am I trying to do this? Well, it goes back to ideas I had a long time ago, and they're not original with me, either. The simplest thought involves the coordination of activity among a large number of widely distributed and specialized brain systems."

In fact, Gevins's idea goes back to the late 1800s and John Hughlings Jackson. A neurologist in the nineteenth century, Jackson made a fundamental observation about the brain and the way it works. Gevins explains it with a TV analogy. "You are looking at a show on a TV set," he says, "and someone takes a little integrated circuit out of the set. The picture turns to stripes. Now, you can't hold up that integrated circuit and say, 'This is the source of "pictureness." ' Yes, it is a critical node in the circuit which produces the picture. But it's not the *location* of 'pictureness.'

"Now, think about that analogy and about how people thought about the brain. It's completely analogous, especially about thinking. You can localize the visual system in the brain, and you can localize feature extractors. You can localize the input and output for language—we have pictures of language, and we can point to Wernicke's and Broca's areas and all that. But thought involves the integration of activity over a large number of widely distributed specialized systems. So it's a network."

In other words, the brain is made of a set of interconnected "modules." Since the early 1980s, Gevins and his colleagues at the EEG Systems Laboratory have been busy measuring signs of communication among those different neural networks in the brain. They use their new-generation EEG machines along with MRI to create detailed structural images of the brain. Says Gevins, "We've taken a very old signal, the EEG, and figured out how to extract a lot more information out of it. And we're using it to try and measure how the brain thinks.

"I figure that everything has already been said about consciousness and thinking and all the rest of that; I just need to get some real measurements."

To do that, to get those measurements, Gevins and his associates have carried out seven major experiments since the late 1970s. Their aim has been to look at the instantaneous neural networks of the brain's association cortex while people are doing some simple tests—simple but complete.

The tests Gevins devised have all the essential aspects of a real full-blown behavior. First comes a preparation interval, Gevins explains, when the subject gets ready to do a specific task. This sets up a mood of anticipation in the subject. Next comes a specific stimulus. The subject must make a decision and carry out a specific action in response to that decision. Finally, people get some feedback about how accurately they responded. That means Gevins can look at the brain updating itself with information about response accuracy. "So these are model behaviors," Gevins says. "They typically last about four seconds. We've got a bunch of experiments like this. Get ready, see something, figure it out, act, and get feedback about what you did."

The more than twenty years that Gevins has been exploring the brain and its thoughts have given him plenty of real measurements. "But for me, the single most amazing thing that has come out of all these experiments," he says, "is how much of the brain's activity is concerned with performing what I call, for lack of better terms, 'high-fidelity real-time simulations of a world and the self.' " That is, a great deal of the brain's activities have to do with making internal models or simulations of what is happening in the outside world and of who we think we are.

"This is not some big philosophical overview I'm giving you," Gevins adds. "This is in every brain system; it's everywhere. I see little signs of these models, little glimpses of them."

THE DANCER AND THE DANCE

The vast majority of brain researchers and other scientists today believe that the mind is not some entity separate from the brain. The consensus seems to be that the mind is what the human brain creates when it's working normally.

We might imagine the connection between mind and brain to be similar to the relationship between a dancer and the dance. The dance is what the dancer does when she is moving in a particular fashion. Crawling is not dancing. Walking is not dancing. Neither is running, jumping, or rolling down a grassy hillside. These are all body movements, and we have all done them at one time or another. But a dancer takes the kinds of body movements we all make, or can make, and combines them in a particularly rhythmic fashion. The rhythms may be ones with which we are culturally familiar—as Americans and Europeans, for example, would find the movements of classical Western ballet. They may also be strange or even jarring, such as those of Japanese Kabuki. Whether familiar or strange, the rhythms exist and are real. But the dance is not the individual movements the dancer makes. It is the entire combination of the movements, in rhythmic patterns, as the dancer moves his or her body through space and time. The dancer may be wearing an elaborate costume or ceremonial clothing, tights and a sweatshirt, or nothing at all. The clothing or lack thereof does not create the dance but may well contribute to its creation and continuing existence.

The dancer may also not be a soloist; she may have a partner or be accompanied by an entire company of other dancers, male and female. Each of the dancers has his or her set of movements. The dance, then, is more than the movements of the individual dancers; it is now the combined movements of them all, in synchrony and counterpoint to one another. Some of the dancers may be improvising their movements, swiftly seeking and finding a particular set of rhythmic movements that match or counterpoint the movements of those around them. Thus, the dance gains still another level of complexity and structure.

There is an old African saying: "If you can talk, you can sing; if you can walk, you can dance." Indeed, even if you can't walk, you can dance. People in wheelchairs can dance as well as anyone. So perhaps most, if not all, people can dance; but the dance cannot exist apart from the dancer. There is no way one can separate the dance from the dancer, in some reductionistic fashion, and then point to it like a surgeon who has removed a spleen from an injured patient and say, "This is dance."

When we think of the mind in this way, we can get an inkling of how something can be real but not material in the accepted sense of that word. Dance is not a material thing the way, say, the body is a material thing. The body is made up of nerves and muscle, bone and skin, blood and connective tissue. These building blocks of the body are made of molecules that are made of atoms that in turn are made of protons, neutrons, and electrons. Dance is constructed from none of these material pieces.

In the same way, the brain is composed of nerves and blood cells and other tissue. The mind, though, is not made up of molecules, atoms, electrons, or quarks. Like dance, it is real but nonmaterial. It is an "emergent property" of the living, working human brain. The mind *emerges* from the brain's electrochemical activities the way dance emerges from a dancer's movements; it rises up like a bright flame from the combustion of the brain's furiously heated action. When the combustion stops, the flame disappears. When the dancer stops moving and, exhausted, sits down and takes off her shoes, the dance ends.

In the same way, the mind cannot exist apart from the living human brain. It is the dance, but the brain is the dancer. Where does the flame go when the campfire is quenched? It doesn't *go* anywhere. It simply stops *being*. Where does the dance go when the dancer finishes? Again, it goes nowhere. It is over, is all. But as long as the brain is alive and functioning above some still-unclear level of activity, the human mind is real and present.

THE MYSTERY OF THE MIND

The leading researchers in this Decade of the Brain are not indifferent to the nature of the mind and its connection to the brain. The very experiments they do, the very results they see painted in phosphor dots on their computer screens, lead them to consider the same questions that philosophers and theologians have been asking for centuries.

When I asked Marcus Raichle, "What is mind? How do you define it, and how do you define consciousness?" he chuckled a little but didn't hesitate to respond. "The mere fact that you're asking the question," he said, "is symptomatic of what's happening in neuroscience. It is now becoming a legitimate question to ask. It used to be a philosophical question, or if you got very late in your career as a neuroscientist, you could talk about it." Raichle was no doubt thinking of Wilder Penfield, the great American-Canadian brain surgeon. His years of work with epileptic patients and his probes of their living brains led him to ponder deeply the relationship between mind and brain. Near the end of his life, Penfield worked on his final book, *The Mystery of the Mind*. He was convinced that scientific study of the brain would indeed finally lead to an understanding of the mind. But as he continued to write and to think, he became less and less sure of that position. Those doubts remained until his death at age eighty-four.

Raichle continued: "There are all sorts of issues about definitions, but I think the vast majority of people without a doubt now believe that [the mind is] a product of the brain. Whether it's related to systems in the brain or the way the brain organizes itself are issues that should be seriously considered.

"Is the mind a manifestation of the brain's intentional system that we are conscious?" Raichle asked. "I was recently at a meeting in Stockholm which brought literary people and brain people together, and it was marvelously fun." One of the topics discussed at the Stockholm meeting, said Raichle, was the contention that a large part of what we do is *not* conscious.

"Think about the conversation that you and I are having right now," said Raichle. "You're not thinking about the individual words, nor am I. And that's just a teeny example of this idea, one that helps us to realize how we automate so much of what we do and then touch it with our conscious behavior. These are important issues as we begin to try to figure out what is the neurobiological substrate of all of this, but they do begin to constrain the problem.

"And I don't doubt that we are eventually going to have a better idea of the nature of the mind."

It is a sunny day in San Francisco. My wife, Judy, explores the shops in the lobby of the Rincon Building, while I sit in the EEG Systems Laboratory conference room across the table from Alan Gevins. He has been showing me colorized computer images of human brain activity measured with his souped-up EEG. The images show different neural networks in the brain as they work, in near real time.

And according to Gevins, they show something even more important.

"This is direct evidence from the brain of the formation of an internal model of self and external reality," says Gevins. "Remember the ancient Greek philosopher Heraclitus?" I do. Heraclitus lived in the early sixth and late fifth centuries BCE and taught that there is no permanent reality except the reality of change. It was Heraclitus who supposedly noted that you cannot step into the same river twice. "Well," Gevins continues, "here's evidence that Heraclitus was right. In essence, the world is being created in the brain."

Gevins admits that this is a somewhat speculative statement. If anyone went looking for this kind of conclusion in his published papers, they would be unlikely to find it. But he sometimes adds a little diagram at the end of his review papers, a diagram he calls "the synthesis of experience."

"As I said before," Gevins explains, "in our brains we humans are running a high-fidelity, real-time simulation of what's going on outside and of who we think we are, where we think we are, what we think is important, all of that. Based upon this simulation or internal model, the same stimulus can be perceived in a completely different manner by the same person over time or by different people in different situations.

"The world we perceive is literally created in the mind of the brain. And we are starting to be able to measure signals of this."

I look at him cautiously, perhaps a bit skeptically. I say, "But we all have a certain amount of agreement on what's 'out there.' When you and I both look at that building across the street, we are both going to say those bricks are red, those panels are black. We can describe the shape of that railing up there, and we agree on that. So there is a similarity of the internal models and of the way that our mind is creating the outside world."

Gevins nods. "Of course. Some of that similarity comes through hardwiring of the brain—for example, the way visual stimuli are broken down. But most of it comes through socialization. I'm sure that you remember the study of a very isolated group of native people who lived in New Guinea who were shown photographs for the first time. The photographs had no meaning to them. That's an example of the effect of socialization on perception."

I understand his point. It reminds me of the experience that the famous British neuropsychologist Richard Gregory had with a man born blind. After an otherwise normal lifetime, the man had an opportunity to undergo an experimental operation that would allow him to actually see for the first time. He took the chance, and the operation worked. But not the way either the man or Gregory expected. The man had been a successful woodworker, for example, and could instantly identify any woodworking tools by touch. But not by sight. When Gregory showed him a wood-turning lathe enclosed in a clear glass box, the man had no idea what it was. When Gregory removed the box and the man closed his eyes and touched it, he at once knew what it was. After a few months of euphoria at being able to see, the man fell into a deep depression. He retired to a darkened room, rarely coming outside anymore. Nothing looked the way he had *thought* it would look, he complained. Within two years of the operation he died, depressed and brokenhearted.

Gevins doesn't know the incident, but he knows what it's about. "The electromagnetic radiation that's hitting our retinas is the same, and a lot of the breaking down of that pattern by our primary visual cortex into features is the same," he says. "But how those patterns are assembled into objects that have *specific meaning*, that's socially learned. If you wanted to focus your will and your concentration and stare at the bricks and turn them into something completely else in your mind, you could."

I raise my eyebrows. This does sound a bit New Agey, but I continue. "What's next for you?" I ask him.

Gevins looks at me with a hint of surprise, perhaps impatience. "Well, it's kind of obvious what we should do next. I think we have the only technology that can measure the brain functioning in the real world. So we're going to go look at people like jet pilots and maybe football quarterbacks. We've already done a race-car driver going over one hundred miles an hour on a racetrack. It was the first time anyone had ever seen the brain activity of someone in a situation like that. So that's what we're going try to do. We going to try and see things that have never been seen before.

"I don't know what we're going to find from that," he continues. "We've created this new instrument"—Gevins's souped-up EEG—"and we're going to have to figure out what to do with it. But you can see how important it is to actually get these measurements out of the laboratory. You can't see the real brain in action if someone's got needles in their arms and they're sitting inside of this brain scanner that's like a very noisy gun barrel. You can only go so far in studying the brain that way because the situation is not real. It's completely artificial."

In the distance we hear the rumble of jet engines. The U.S. Navy's famed Blue Angels are flying over San Francisco Bay, practicing for an upcoming air show. The noise occasionally drowns out our conversation. Gevins pauses until the sound diminishes. "The guys who fly those Blue Angels planes? I was once watching them with binoculars, and they were *so good*! And I was thinking to myself, What is going on in their minds?

"And then I realized that I could make a technology that would measure it. That was a few years ago. Since that time, we developed everything we need."

Gevins pauses and smiles. "I'm real interested in the mind itself," he says, "in that high-fidelity, real-time internal model. Real interested."

APPENDIX A
HOUSE JOINT RESOLUTION 174

DECADE OF THE BRAIN

PUBLIC LAW 101-58
101ST CONGRESS
JULY 25, 1989
H. J. RES. 174

Joint Resolution to designate the decade beginning January 1, 1990, as the "Decade of the Brain."

Whereas it is estimated that fifty million Americans are affected each year by disorders and disabilities that involve the brain, including the major mental illnesses; inherited and degenerative diseases; stroke; epilepsy; addictive disorders; injury resulting from prenatal events, environmental neurotoxins and trauma; and speech, language, hearing and other cognitive disorders;

Whereas it is estimated that treatment, rehabilitation and related costs of disorders and disabilities that affect the brain represents a total economic burden of $305,000,000,000 annually;

Whereas the people of the Nation should be aware of the exciting research advances on the brain and of the availability of effective treatment of disorders and disabilities that affect the brain;

Whereas a technological revolution occurring in the brain sciences, resulting in such procedures as positron emission tomography and magnetic resonance imaging, permits clinical researchers to observe the living brain noninvasively and in exquisite detail, to define brain systems that are implicated in specific disorders and disabilities, to study complex neuropeptides and behavior as well as to begin to learn about the complex structures underlying memory;

Whereas scientific information on the brain is amassing at an enormous rate, and the field of computer and information sciences has reached a level of sophistication sufficient to handle neuroscience data in a manner that would be maximally useful to both basic researchers and clinicians dealing with brain function and dysfunction;

Whereas advances in mathematics, physics, computational science, and brain imaging technologies have made possible the initiation of significant work in imaging brain function and pathology, modeling neural networks and simulating their dynamic interactions;

Whereas comprehending the reality of the nervous system is still on the frontier of technological innovation requiring a comprehensive effort to decipher how individual neurons, by their collective action, give rise to human intelligence;

Whereas fundamental discoveries at the molecular and cellular levels of the organization of the brain are clarifying the role of the brain in translating neurophysiologic events into behavior, thought, and emotion;

Whereas molecular biology and molecular genetics have yielded strategies effective in preventing several forms of severe mental retardation and are contributing to promising breakthroughs in the study of inheritable neurological disorders, such as Huntington's disease, and mental disorders, such as affective illnesses;

Whereas the capacity to map the biochemical circuitry of neurotransmitters and neuromodulators will permit the rational design of potent medications possessing minimal adverse effects that will act on the discrete neurochemical deficits associated with such disorders as Parkinson's disease, schizophrenia and Alzheimer's disease;

Whereas the incidence of neurologic, psychiatric, psychological, and cognitive disorders and disabilities exprienced by older persons will increase in the future as the number of older persons increases;

Whereas studies of the brain and central nervous system will contribute not only to the relief of neurologic, psychiatric, psychological, and cognitive disorders, but also to the management of fertility and infertility, cardiovascular disease, infectious and parasitic diseases, developmental disabilities and immunologic disorders, as well as to an understanding of behavioral factors that underlie the leading preventable causes of death in this Nation;

Whereas the central nervous and immune systems are both signalling systems which serve the entire organism, and there are direct connections between the nervous and immune systems, and whereas studies of the modulatory effects of each system on the other will enhance our understanding of diseases as diverse as the major psychiatric disorders, acquired immune deficiency syndrome, and autoimmune disorders;

Whereas recent discoveries have led to fundamental insights as to why people abuse drugs, how abused drugs affect brain function leading to addiction, and how some of these drugs cause permanent brain damage;

Whereas studies of the brain will contribute to the development of new treatments that will curtail the craving for drugs, break the addictive effects of drugs, prevent the brain-mediated "high" caused by certain abused drugs, and lessen the damage done to the developing minds of babies, who are the innocent victims of drug abuse;

Whereas treatment for persons with head injury, developmental disabilities, speech, hearing, and other cognitive functions is increasing in availability and effectiveness;

Whereas the study of the brain involves the multidisciplinary efforts of scientists from such diverse areas as physiology, biochemistry, psychology, psychiatry, molecular biology, anatomy, medicine, genetics, and many others working together toward the common goals of better understanding the structure of the brain and how it affects our development, health, and behavior;

Whereas the Nobel Prize for Medicine or Physiology has been awarded to fifteen neuroscientists within the past twenty-five years, an achievement that underscores the excitement and productivity of the study of the brain and central nervous system and its potential for contributing to the health of humanity;

Whereas the people of the Nation should be concerned with research into disorders and disabilities that affect the brain, and should recognize prevention and treatment of such disorders and disabilities as a health priority; and

Whereas the declaration of the Decade of the Brain will focus needed government attention on research, treatment, and rehabilitation in this area: Now, therefore, be it

Resolved by the Senate and House of Representatives of the United States of America in Congress assembled, That the decade beginning January 1, 1990, hereby is designated "Decade of the Brain," and the President of the United States is authorized and requested to issue a proclamation calling upon all public officials and the people of the United States to observe such decade with appropriate programs and activities.

Congressional Record, Vol. 135 (1989):

June 29, considered and passed House.

July 13, considered and passed Senate.

APPENDIX B
IMPORTANT RADIOACTIVE ISOTOPES

An isotope is one of several "flavors" of any particular element. To be more scientific, isotopes are atoms of the same element that vary in atomic weight or mass number. The word comes from the Greek *iso*, meaning "identical" or "the same," and *topos*, "place."

Some isotopes may be stable and remain unchanged for hundreds of billions of years. Other isotopes are unstable, or radioactive; they release various subatomic particles, or bursts of energy, and eventually decay into a stable form of another element. A radioisotope has a specific lifetime that is referred to as its *half-life*. A radioactive element's half-life is the time it takes for half of the atoms in a specific sample of that element to decay into its final stable form.

Subatomic particles called protons and neutrons constitute an atom's inner core or nucleus. The atom's number of protons is called its atomic number. Electrons occupy a series of "shells" or regions farther out from the nucleus. A proton has a positive charge equal to the negative charge of an electron. In any atom, the number of protons and electrons is equal. Neutrons have no electric charge. The number of neutrons can vary in atoms of the same element but has no effect on either the number of electrons or the atom's atomic number. The total number of protons and electrons in an atom's nucleus equals its mass number.

An element's chemical properties are determined by its electrons, because all chemical reactions are caused by interactions between the electrons in the outermost regions of different atoms. However, differences in the composition of the nucleus can have some slight effects on other properties of an atom. In particular, the number of neutrons in an atomic nucleus can affect the weight of the nucleus and therefore of the atom.

Take carbon as an example. Carbon has several different isotopes. Two are stable, or nonradioactive, isotopes and are known as carbon 12 and carbon 13. Carbon 14 is a radioactive isotope with six protons and eight neutrons—an atomic number of 6, like all atoms of carbon, and a mass number of 14. Carbon 14 has a half-life of 5,730 years. This means that in a sample of a million atoms of carbon 14, half of them will have decayed into nitrogen 14 after 5,730 years. After another 5,730 years, half of the remaining carbon 14 (250,000 atoms) will have decayed to nitrogen 14. And so on.

Several of the most important brain-imaging technologies, including PET and SPECT, are actually offshoots of nuclear medicine. Nuclear medicine uses radioactive forms of certain elements, called radioactive isotopes or radioisotopes, to diagnose and treat certain illnesses. Nuclear medicine is a common part of some cancer therapy, for example.

In the early 1970s, researchers like Marcus Raichle and Michael Phelps at Washington University (Phelps is now at UCLA) realized that the mathematical and computer techniques that made CT scanning possible could be adapted to nuclear medicine. Radioisotopes could be used to image the activity of certain organs of the body, including the brain, and produce functional maps. Since the development of the first PET scanner and the refinement of SPECT scanning, several radioisotopes have become common in this new field of medical imaging. Here's some basic information on some of these important radioisotopes.

CARBON 11

Carbon (C) is element number 6 on the Periodic Table and has been known to humanity since prehistoric times. (The name comes from the Latin word meaning "charcoal.") Carbon is an essential component of all living organisms. The two stable isotopes are carbon 12 and carbon 13. More than 98 percent of the carbon on Earth is carbon 12; carbon 13 comprises practically all the rest. Carbon 14 is the best-known radioactive isotope of carbon and has a half-life of 5,730 years. It is used in carbon dating of old organic material. Carbon 11, by contrast, has a half-life of about twenty minutes, and is thus a good radioisotope for use in medical imaging. The other isotopes of carbon, and their half-lives, are:

Name	Half-Life
carbon 8	1.9827×10^{-21} seconds
carbon 9	0.1265 seconds
carbon 10	19.255 seconds
carbon 15	2.449 seconds
carbon 16	0.747 seconds
carbon 17	0.193 seconds
carbon 18	0.066 seconds

FLUORINE 18

Element 9 on the Periodic Table, fluorine (F) is a light yellow gas at room temperature. It was discovered in 1886 in France by Henri Moissan. Its name derives from French and Latin words meaning "flow" or "flux." Fluorine 19 is the most common and only stable isotope of this element. Fluorine 18 is a radioactive isotope with a half-life of 1.829 hours, or about 109 minutes, and it is often used in PET scan experiments with the human brain. The other isotopes of fluorine are:

Name	Half-Life
fluorine 15	4.652×10^{-22} seconds
fluorine 16	1.1406×10^{-21} seconds
fluorine 17	1.0748 minutes
fluorine 20	11.00 seconds
fluorine 21	4.158 seconds
fluorine 22	4.23 seconds
fluorine 23	2.223 seconds
fluorine 24	0.34 seconds
fluorine 27	?

GALLIUM 68

Gallium (Ga, element 31 on the Periodic Table) was discovered in France in 1875 by Paul Emile Lecoq de Boisbaudran. At room temperature it is a silvery white liquid. (The name "gallium" comes from the Latin word *Gallia,* for France. It is also no coincidence that the Latin word *gallus* is a translated form of de Boisbaudran's middle name *Lecoq,* or rooster.) The two most common isotopes of gallium are gallium 69 and gallium 71. The former makes up about 60 percent of the gallium on Earth, while the latter constitutes the rest. Gallium 68 has a half-life of 1.127 hours, or about 67 minutes. Twenty-six different isotopes or versions of gallium have been discovered or created. Except for the two stable forms, none has a half-life longer than three days.

NITROGEN 13

Nitrogen (N, element 7 on the Periodic Table) is the most common element in the earth's atmosphere, which is about 80 percent nitrogen and 20 percent oxygen. Daniel Rutherford of Scotland discovered nitrogen in 1772 and derived its name from the Latin word for "soda" and the Greek word for "forming" or "making." The two stable isotopes of nitrogen are nitrogen 14 (99 percent of all nitrogen) and nitrogen 15. Nitrogen 13 has a half-life of 9.9 minutes and is a common radioisotope in nuclear medicine. The other radioactive forms of nitrogen are:

Name	Half-Life
nitrogen 10	10.4 minutes
nitrogen 11	?
nitrogen 12	0.011 seconds
nitrogen 16	7.13 seconds
nitrogen 16m	5.25×10^{-6} seconds
nitrogen 17	4.173 seconds
nitrogen 18	0.624 seconds
nitrogen 19	0.27 seconds
nitrogen 20	0.1 seconds

OXYGEN 15

Together with nitrogen, oxygen (O, element 8 on the Periodic Table) comprises the bulk of the Earth's atmosphere. Oxygen is essential for nearly all life on Earth. Discovered by Karl Wilhelm Scheele in Sweden in 1772 and independently in England by Joseph Priestley in 1774, the name comes from the Greek prefix meaning "sharp" or "acid." Its three stable isotopes are oxygen 16, oxygen 17, and oxygen 18. More than 99 percent of all oxygen is oxygen 16. The radioactive isotope oxygen 15 has a half-life of a little over two minutes. It is widely used as a tracer for PET scans and in this role has contributed to a vast revolution in our understanding of how the human brain works. The other known isotopes of oxygen include:

Name	Half-Life
oxygen 12	1.1406×10^{-21} seconds
oxygen 13	0.0085 seconds
oxygen 14	70.608 seconds
oxygen 19	26.91 seconds
oxygen 20	13.51 seconds
oxygen 21	3.42 seconds
oxygen 22	2.25 seconds
oxygen 23	0.082 seconds
oxygen 24	0.061 seconds

RUBIDIUM 82

Rubidium (Rb) is element 37 on the Periodic Table. It was discovered by Robert Bunson and Gustav Kirchhoff in 1861; the name comes from a Latin word meaning "deepest red." At room temperature, rubidium is a soft, silvery white solid. However, rubidium is highly reactive and ignites spontaneously in air. Rubidium 85 is the only stable isotope, and constitutes about 72 percent of the earth's rubidium. The rest of it is rubidium 87, a naturally occurring radioactive isotope with a half-life of over 47 billion years. The radioactive decay of rubidium 87 into strontium 87 is the basis of the rubidium-strontium method for dating very old geologic formations. Rubidium 82 has a half-life of 1.27 hours, or 76 minutes, making it useful for SPECT scanning. A total of 38 different isotopes of rubidium have been discovered or created. Other than rubidium 85 and rubidium 87, they all have half-lives of less than three months.

TECHNITIUM 99

Technitium (Tc, element 43 on the Periodic Table) is a radioactive element that does not occur naturally on Earth. It was created in 1937 by Emilio Segre and Carlo Perrier of Italy; the name comes from the Greek word meaning "artificial." The most stable isotope is technitium 99, which has a half-life of 2.6 million years. At room temperature, the element is a silvery-gray solid. Thirty-eight different isotopes or variations of technitium have been created. A version of technitium 99 called technitium 99m has a half-life of about six hours. This makes it emininently suitable for use in SPECT scanning. The other isotopes have half-lives ranging from about a millionth of a second to 61 days.

Thallium 201

Thallium (T1, element 81 on the Periodic Table) is a grayish metallic element that occurs naturally on Earth in very small quantities, usually in iron or zinc ores. It was discovered in 1861 by Sir William Crookes. (Its name derives from the Greek work meaning "a green shoot" or "twig.") Thallium 203 and thallium 205 are stable isotopes, with thallium 205 accounting for almost 71 percent of all the element. Thallium 201, with a half-life of about three days, is used in some SPECT imaging experiments. Fifty-four different isotopes of thallium have been either discovered or created. Most are radioactive and have short half-lives.

APPENDIX C:
THE PERIODIC TABLE OF ELEMENTS

Legend: Metals | Metalloids | Nonmetals

IA	IIA	IIIB	IVB	VB	VIB	VIIB	VIII	VIII	VIII	IB	IIB	IIIA	IVA	VA	VIA	VIIA	0
1 H 1.0079																1 H 1.0079	2 He 4.0026
3 Li 6.941	4 Be 9.0122											5 B 10.811	6 C 12.011	7 N 14.0067	8 O 15.9994	9 F 18.9984	10 Ne 20.1797
11 Na 22.9898	12 Mg 24.3050											13 Al 26.9815	14 Si 28.0855	15 P 30.9738	16 S 32.066	17 Cl 35.4527	18 Ar 39.948
19 K 39.0983	20 Ca 40.078	21 Sc 44.9559	22 Ti 47.88	23 V 50.9415	24 Cr 51.9961	25 Mn 54.9380	26 Fe 55.847	27 Co 58.9332	28 Ni 58.69	29 Cu 63.546	30 Zn 65.39	31 Ga 69.723	32 Ge 72.61	33 As 74.9216	34 Se 78.96	35 Br 79.904	36 Kr 83.80
37 Rb 85.4678	38 Sr 87.62	39 Y 88.9059	40 Zr 91.224	41 Nb 92.9064	42 Mo 95.94	43 Tc (98)	44 Ru 101.07	45 Rh 102.9055	46 Pd 106.42	47 Ag 107.8682	48 Cd 112.411	49 In 114.82	50 Sn 118.710	51 Sb 121.75	52 Te 127.60	53 I 126.9045	54 Xe 131.29
55 Cs 132.9054	56 Ba 137.327	57 *La 138.9055	72 Hf 178.49	73 Ta 180.9479	74 W 183.85	75 Re 186.207	76 Os 190.2	77 Ir 192.22	78 Pt 195.08	79 Au 196.9665	80 Hg 200.59	81 Tl 204.3833	82 Pb 207.2	83 Bi 208.9804	84 Po (209)	85 At (210)	86 Rn (222)
87 Fr (223)	88 Ra (226)	89 **Ac (227)	104 Unq (261)	105 Unp (262)	106 Unh (263)	107 Uns (262)	108	109									

*Lanthanide Series

58 Ce 140.115	59 Pr 140.9076	60 Nd 144.24	61 Pm (145)	62 Sm 150.36	63 Eu 151.965	64 Gd 157.25	65 Tb 158.9253	66 Dy 162.50	67 Ho 164.9303	68 Er 167.26	69 Tm 168.9342	70 Yb 173.04	71 Lu 174.967

**Actinide Series

90 Th 232.0381	91 Pa 231.0359	92 U 238.0289	93 Np (237)	94 Pu (244)	95 Am (243)	96 Cm (247)	97 Bk (247)	98 Cf (251)	99 Es (252)	100 Fm (257)	101 Md (258)	102 No (259)	103 Lr (260)

Note: Atomic masses are 1987 IUPAC values (up to four decimal places).

263

BIBLIOGRAPHY

The following list of books, magazine articles, and research papers is not intended to be a comprehensive overview of the Decade of the Brain or current neurobiology. However, it does include most of the source material for this book. Not all the information in all the sources listed ended up in the book. But for those who wish to either look at primary sources or browse the field more extensively, this list may prove useful.

BOOKS

Brain Facts: A Primer on the Brain and Nervous System. Washington, D.C.: Society for Neuroscience, 1993.
Computational Models of Visual Processes. Cambridge, Mass.: MIT Press, 1991.
Crick, Francis. *The Astonishing Hypothesis: The Scientific Search for the Soul.* New York: Scribners, 1993.
Eccles, Sir John, ed. *Mind and Brain: The Many-Faceted Problems.* Washington, D.C.: Paragon House, 1982.
Edelman, Gerald H. *Bright Air, Brilliant Fire: On the Matter of the Mind.* New York: Basic Books, 1992.
Falk, Dean. *Braindance: New Discoveries About Human Origins and Brain Evolution.* New York: Henry Holt, 1992.
Fischler, Martin A., and Oscar Firschein. *Intelligence: The Eye, the Brain, and the Computer.* Reading, Mass.: Addison-Wesley, 1987.
Gazzaniga, Michael S. *Mind Matters: How the Mind & Brain Interact to Create Our Conscious Lives.* Boston: Houghton Mifflin, 1988.
_____. *Nature's Mind: The Biological Roots of Thinking, Emotions, Sexuality, Language, and Intelligence.* New York: Basic Books, 1992.
_____. *The Social Brain: Discovering the Networks of the Mind.* New York: Basic Books, 1985.
Herbert, Nick. *Elemental Mind: Human Consciousness and the New Physics.* New York: Penguin Books, 1993.
Humphrey, Nicholas. *A History of the Mind: Evolution and the Birth of Consciousness.* New York: Simon & Schuster, 1992.

Kingdon, Jonathan. *Self-Made Man: Human Evolution From Eden to Extinction.* New York: John Wiley, 1993.

Kosslyn, Stephen M., and Olivier Koenig. *Wet Mind: The New Cognitive Neuroscience.* New York: Free Press, 1992.

LeDoux, Joseph E., and William Hirst, eds. *Mind and Brain: Dialogues on Cognitive Neuroscience.* New York: Cambridge University Press, 1986.

Levine, Daniel S. *Introduction to Neural and Cognitive Modeling.* Hillsdale, N.J.: Lawrence Erlbaum Associates, 1991.

Nadeau, Robert. *Mind, Machines, and Human Consciousness.* Chicago: Contemporary Books, 1991.

Ornstein, Robert. *The Roots of the Self: Unraveling the Mystery of Who We Are.* San Francisco: HarperSanFrancisco, 1992.

Pool, Robert. *The Dynamic Brain.* Washington, D.C.: National Academy Press, 1994.

U.S. Congress. Office of Technology Assessment. *Neural Grafting: Repairing the Brain and Spinal Cord.* OTA-BA-462. Washington, D.C.: U.S. Government Printing Office. September 1990.

_____. *The Biology of Mental Disorders.* OTA-BA-538. Washington, DC: U.S. Government Printing Office, September 1992.

Zohar, Dana. *The Quantum Self: Human Nature and Consciousness Defined by the New Physics.* New York: William Morrow, 1990.

ARTICLES

Adler, Tina. "Comprehending Those Who Can't Relate." *Science News* (April 1994): 248–49.

Allison, Malorye. "Stopping the Brain Drain." *Harvard Health Letter* (October 1991): 6–9.

Allmann, William F. "The Mental Edge." *U.S. News & World Report* (August 3, 1992): 50–56.

"The Anatomy of Memory Loss." *Science News* (September 23, 1989): 204.

Angier, Natalie. "Powerhouse of Senses, Smell, at Last Gets Its Due." *New York Times* (February 14, 1995): C1, C6.

Assad, John A., and John H. R. Maunsell. "Neuronal Correlates of Inferred Motion in Primate Posterior Parietal Cortex." *Nature* 373 (February 9, 1995): 518–21.

Bailey, Craig H., and Eric R. Kandel. "Structural Changes Accompanying Memory Storage." In *Annual Review of Physiology*, edited by Joseph F. Hoffman. Palo Alto, Calif: Annual Review, Inc., 1993, 397–426.

Barinaga, Marcia. "How Scary Things Get That Way." *Science* 258 (November 6, 1992): 887–88.

_____. "How the Nose Knows: Olfactory Receptor Cloned." *Science* 252 (April 12, 1991): 209–10.

_____. "The Brain Remaps Its Own Contours." *Science* 258 (October 9, 1992): 216–18.

_____. "The Remembrance of Blinks Past." *Science* 260 (May 14, 1993): 234–36.

_____. "The Tide of Memory, Turning." *Science* 248 (June 29, 1990): 1603–5.

_____. "To Sleep, Perchance To . . . Learn? New Studies Say Yes." *Science* 265 (July 29, 1994): 603–4.

_____. "Watching the Brain Remake Itself." *Science* 266 (December 2, 1994): 1475–76.

Beardsley, Tim. "Commanding Attention." *Scientific American* (February 1995): 16.

_____. "Molecular Mischief." *Scientific American* (March 1994): 20–1.

Begley, Sharon. "Mapping the Brain." *Newsweek* (April 20, 1992): 66–70.

"Behaviorism, Cognitivism and the Neuropsychology of Memory." *American Scientist* (January 1994): 30–37.

Behrmann, Marlene, Gordon Winocur, and Morris Moscovitch. "Dissociation Between Mental Imagery and Object Recognition in a Brain-Damaged Patient." *Nature* 359 (October 15, 1992): 636–37.

"The Biological Significance of Iron-Related Magnetic Resonance Imaging Changes in the Brain." Abstract. In *Journal of the American Medical Association* 268, no. 23 (December 16, 1992): 3309.

Bishop, Jerry. "The Knowing Eye: One Man's Accident Is Shedding New Light on Human Perception." *Wall Street Journal* (September 30, 1993): A1, A8.

_____. "Word Processing: Stroke Patients Yield Clues to Brain's Ability to Create Language." *Wall Street Journal* (October 13, 1994): A1, A14.

Black, Pamela J. "No One's Sniffing at Aroma Research Now." *Business Week* (December 23, 1991): 82–83.

Blakeslee, Sandra. "Brain Yields New Clues on Its Organization for Language." *New York Times* (September 10, 1991): C1, C8.

_____. "Evolution of Tabby Cat Mapped in Brain Study." *New York Times* (January 12, 1993): C1, C8.

_____. "Scanner Pinpoints Site of Thoughts As Brain Sees or Speaks." *New York Times* (June 1, 1993): B5–B6.

_____. "Scientists Find Place on Left Side of the Brain Where Perfect Pitch Is Heard." *New York Times* (February 3, 1995): A16.

_____. "Seeing and Imagining: Clues to the Workings of the Mind's Eye." *New York Times* (August 31, 1993): C1, C7.

_____. "The Mystery of Music: How It Works in the Brain." *New York Times* (May 16, 1995): C1, C10.

Bower, Bruce. "A Few Words From the Brain." *Science News* 145 (May 28, 1994): 347.

———. "Babies' Brains Charge Up to Speech Sounds." *Science News* 146 (July 30, 1994): 71.

———. "Brain Faces Up to Fear, Social Signs." *Science News* 146 (December 17, 1994): 406.

———. "Brain Images Delve into Hyperactivity." *Science News* 145 (May 14, 1994): 309.

———. "Brain Images Reveal Cerebral Side of Music." *Science News* 145 (April 23, 1994): 261.

———. "Brain Images Reveal Key Language Areas." *Science News* 138 (September 1, 1990): 134.

———. "Brain Images Show Structure of Depression." *Science News* 142 (September 12, 1992): 165.

———. "Brain Scans Show Two-Sided Memory Flow." *Science News* 145 (March 26, 1994): 199.

———. "Brain Scans Tag Sexes as Words Apart." *Science News* 147 (February 19, 1995): 101.

———. "Brain Study Finds Possible Word Center." *Science News* 146 (November 19, 1994): 325.

———. "Chicks Hatch Chemical Clues to Memory." *Science News* 143 (April 17, 1993): 244.

———. "Child Sexual Abuse: Sensory Recall." *Science News* 145 (June 4, 1994): 365.

———. "Clues to the Brain's Knowledge Systems." *Science News* 142 (September 5, 1992): 148.

———. "Conscious Memories May Emerge in Infants." *Science News* 148 (August 5, 1995): 86.

———. "Going With the Flow of Musical Brains." *Science News* 142 (July 11, 1992): 21.

———. "Hormone Shows Link to Some Obsessions." *Science News* 146 (October 29, 1994): 277.

———. "Images of Intellect." *Science News* 146 (October 8, 1994): 236–37.

———. "Infant Memory Shows the Power of Place." *Science News* 141 (April 18, 1992): 244–45.

———. "Language Without Rules." *Science News* 145 (May 28, 1994): 346–47.

———. "Left Brain May Serve as Language Director." *Science News* 141 (March 7, 1992): 149.

———. "Neurons May Take Panoramic View of Sounds." *Science News* 145 (May 7, 1994): 292.

———. "Smoke Gets In Your Brain." *Science News* 143 (January 16, 1993): 46–47.

_____. "The Great Brain Drain." *Science News* 138 (October 13, 1990): 232–34.

Bradley, David C., Ning Qian, and Richard A. Anderson. "Integration of Motion and Steropsis in Middle Temporal Cortical Area of Macaques." *Nature* 373 (February 16, 1995): 609–11.

"Breast-Fed Brains." *Discover* (July 1992): 14–15.

"The Call of the Left Brain." *Science News* 145 (May 21, 1994): 333.

Came, Barry. "Clues in the Brain." *Macleans* (July 19, 1993): 40–41.

"A Cerebral Structure on Magnetic Resonance Imaging in Language- and Learning-Impaired Children." Abstract. In *Journal of the American Medical Association* 266, no. 12 (September 25, 1991): 1636.

Chase, Marilyn. "Inner Music: Imagination May Play Role in How the Brain Learns Muscle Control." *Wall Street Journal* (October 13, 1993): A1, A6.

Christensen, D. "Nursing Mother Rats Show Brain Changes." *Science News* 145 (April 5, 1994): 229–30.

Clarke, John. "SQUIDs." *Scientific American* (August 1994): 47–53.

Collins, Jane. "Female Intuition?" *Lancet* 342 (November 13, 1993): 1188–89.

Connaughton, P. Noel, et al. "Decade of the Brain: A Midpoint Status Report." *Patient Care* (July 15, 1995): 94–114.

Connors, Diane. "Interview: Michael Gazzaniga." *Omni* (October 1993): 99–110.

Coppens, Yves. "East Side Story: The Origin of Humankind." *Scientific American* (May 1994): 88–95.

Corballis, Michael C. "Dividing the Mind." A review of *Brain Asymmetry*, by Richard J. Davidson and Kenneth Hugdahl, MIT Press, 1994. *Nature* (February 2, 1995): 397.

Cotton, Paul. "Neurophysiology, Philosophy on Collision Course?" *Journal of the American Medical Association* 269, no. 12 (March 24, 1993): 1485–86.

_____. "Scientists Chart Course for Brain Map." *Journal of the American Medical Association* 269, no. 11 (March 17, 1993): 1357.

Cowen, Ron. "Brain Gets Thoughtful Reappraisal." *Science News* 146 (October 29, 1994): 284.

_____. "Imaging Clues to Schizophrenia." *Science News* 146 (October 29, 1994): 284.

_____. "In the Valleys of Thought." *Science News* 146 (November 12, 1994): 312.

Cowey, Alan, and Patra Stoerig. "Blindsight in Monkeys." *Nature* 373 (January 19, 1995): 247–49.

Creutzfeldt, O., and G. Ojemann. "Neuronal Activity in the Human Lateral Temporal Lobe. III. Activity Changes During Music." *Experimental Brain Research* 77 (1989): 490–98.

Creutzfeldt, O., G. Ojemann, and E. Lettich. "Neuronal Activity in the Human Lateral Temporal Lobe. I. Responses to Speech." *Experimental Brain Research* 77 (1989): 451–75.

_____. "Neuronal Activity in the Human Lateral Temporal Lobe. II. Responses to the Subject's Own Voice." *Experimental Brain Research* 77 (1989): 476–89.

Crick, Francis, and Christof Koch. "The Problem of Consciousness." *Scientific American* 267, no. 3 (September 1992): 152.

Dajer, Tony. "How the Nose Knows." *Discover* (January 1992): 67.

Damasio, A.R., et al. "Neural Regionalization of Knowledge Access: Preliminary Evidence." In *Cold Spring Harbor Symposia on Quantitative Biology*. vol. 15, Cold Spring Harbor, Me.: Cold Spring Harbor Press, 1990, 1039–47.

Damasio, Antonio. "Synchronous Activation in Multiple Cortical Regions: A Mechanism for Recall." *The Neurosciences* 2 (1990): 287–96.

Damasio, Antonio R. "Aphasia." *New England Journal of Medicine* 326 (February 20, 1992): 531–39.

_____. "Category-Related Recognition Defects as a Clue to the Neural Substrates of Knowledge." *Trends in Neuroscience* 13, no. 3 (March 1990): 95–98.

_____. "Concepts in the Brain." *Mind & Language* 4, no. 1–2 (Spring–Summer 1988): 24–28.

_____. "The Brain Binds Entities and Events by Multiregional Activation From Convergence Zones." *Neural Computation* 1 (1989): 123–32.

_____. "Time-Locked Multiregional Retroactivation: A Systems-Level Proposal for the Neural Substrates of Recall and Recognition." *Cognition* 33, no. 1–2 (1989): 25–62.

Damasio, Antonio R., and Hanna Damasio. "Brain and Language." *Scientific American* (September 1992): 88–95.

Damasio, Antonio R., Daniel Tranel, and Hanna Damasio. "Face Agnosia and the Neural Substrates of Memory." In *Annual Review of Neurosciences*. Palo Alto, Calif: Annual Reviews, Inc., 1990, 89–109.

Damasio, Hanna, and Antonio R. Damasio. "The Neural Basis of Memory, Language and Behavioral Guidance: Advances With the Lesion Method in Humans." *The Neurosciences* 2 (1990): 277–86.

Damasio, Hanna, et al. "The Return of Phineas Gage: Clues About the Brain From the Skull of a Famous Patient." *Science* 264 (May 20, 1994): 1102–5.

Desimone, Robert. "The Physiology of Memory: Recordings of Things Past." *Science* 258 (October 9, 1992): 245–46.

Douglas, Rodney J., and Kevan A. C. Martin. "Vibrations in the Memory." *Nature* 373 (February 16, 1995): 563–64.

Drevets, Wayne C., et al. "Blood Flow Changes in Human Somatosensory Cortex During Anticipated Stimulation." *Nature* 373 (January 19, 1995): 249–52.

Duff, Karen, and John Hardy. "Mouse Model Made." *Nature* 373 (February 9, 1995): 476–77.

Eichenbaum, Howard. "Thinking About Brain Cell Assemblies." *Science* 261 (August 20, 1991): 993–94.

Erickson, Deborah. "Brain Food." *Scientific American* (November 1991): 124, 126.

Ezzell, Carol. "For a Good Memory, Dream On." *Science News* 142 (November 14, 1992): 333.

_____. "Membrane Molecule Guides Nerve Growth." *Science News* 140 (November 23, 1991): 333.

_____. "Monitoring Memories Moving in the Brain." *Science News* 141 (May 2, 1992): 294.

_____. "Receptor Involved in Brain Injury Found." *Science News* 140 (November 23, 1991): 333.

_____. "This Is Your Baby's Brain on Alcohol." *Science News* 142 (November 7, 1992): 317.

_____. "Watching the Remembering Brain at Work." *Science News* 140 (November 23, 1991): 333.

Fackelmann, K. "Mice Show Alzheimer's Brain Plaques." *Science News* 147 (February 11, 1995): 84.

"A False Alarm." *Psychology Today* (October 1993): 24.

Farquharson, James, et. al. "Infant Cerebral Cortex Phospholipid Fatty-Acid Composition and Diet." *Lancet* 340 (October 3, 1992): 810–13.

Finlay, Barbara, and Richard Darlington. "Linked Regularities in the Development and Evolution of Mammalian Brains." *Science* (June 16, 1995): 1578–84.

Fischbach, Gerald D. "Mind and Brain." *Scientific American* 267, no. 3 (September 1992): 48.

Freedman, David H. "Quantum Consciousness." *Discover* (June 1994): 88–98.

Freedman, David H., and Patricia Cadsby. "In the Realm of the Chemical." *Discover* (June 1993): 68.

Friden, Philip M., et al. "Blood-Brain Barrier Penetration and in Vivo Activity of an NGF Conjugate." *Science* 259 (January 15, 1993): 373–77.

Friedman-Hill, Stacia R., et al. "Parietal Contributions to Visual Feature Binding: Evidence From a Patient with Bilateral Lesions." *Science* (August 11, 1995): 853–55.

Games, Dora, et al. "Alzheimer-Type Neuropathology in Transgenic Mice Overexpressing V717F ß-amyloid Precursor Protein." *Nature* 373 (February 9, 1995): 523–27.

Georgopoulos, Apostolos P., et al. "Cognitive Neurophysiology of the Motor Cortex." *Science* 260 (April 2, 1993): 47–52.

Gershon, Eliot S., and Ronald O. Rieder. "Major Disorders of Mind and Brain." *Scientific American* 267, no. 3 (September 1992): 126.

Gevins, Alan S., et al. "Human Neuroelectric Patterns Predict Performance Accuracy." *Science* 235 (January 30, 1987): 580–85.

Gibbons, Ann. "Did Cooler Heads Prevail?" *Science* 250 (December 7, 1990): 1338–39.

_____. "Empathy and Brain Evolution." *Science* 259 (February 26, 1993): 1250–51.

_____. "The Anatomy of Autism." *Discover* (January 1989): 54.

Glanz, James. "Do Chaos Control Techniques Offer Hope for Epilepsy?" *Science* 265 (August 26, 1994): 1174.

Goldman-Rakic, Patricia S. "Working Memory and the Mind." *Scientific American* 267, no. 3 (September 1992): 110.

Goleman, Daniel. "Biologists Find Site of Working Memory." *New York Times* (May 2, 1995): C1, C9.

_____. "New Kind of Memory Found to Preserve Moments of Emotion." *New York Times* (October 25, 1994): C1, C11.

_____. "Provoking a Patient's Worst Fears to Determine the Brain's Role." *New York Times* (June 13, 1995): C1, C10.

_____. "The Brain Manages Happiness and Sadness in Different Centers." *New York Times* (March 28, 1995): C1.

Goode, Erika A. "Where Emotions Come From." *U.S. News & World Report* (June 24, 1991): 54–62.

Gorman, Christine. "How Gender May Bend Your Thinking." *Time* (July 17, 1995): 51.

Greenberg, J. "Early Hearing Loss and Brain Development." *Science News* 131 (March 7, 1987): 149.

Gregory, Richard L. "Seeing Backwards in Time." *Nature* 373 (January 5, 1995): 21–22.

Gurd, Jennifer M., and John C. Marshall. "Drawing Upon the Mind's Eye." *Nature* 359 (October 15, 1992): 590–91.

Hari, Riitta, and Olli V. Lounasmaa. "Recording and Interpretation of Cerebral Magnetic Fields." *Science* 244 (April 28, 1989): 432–36.

Hilchey, Tim. "New Signal Found for Wiring Brain." *New York Times* (July 6, 1993): C3.

Hilts, Philip J. "Brain's Memory System Comes Into Focus." *New York Times* (May 30, 1995): C1, C3.

Hinton, Geoffrey E. "How Neural Networks Learn From Experience." *Scientific American* 267, no. 3 (September 1992): 144.

Holloway, Marguerite. "Under Construction: Temporary Scaffolding Guides Nerves in the Developing Brain." *Scientific American* (January 1992): 25, 27.

Horgan, John. "Can Science Explain Consciousness?" *Scientific American* (July 1994): 88–94.

_____. "Neural Eavesdropping." *Scientific American* (May 1994): 16.

_____. "Quantum Consciousness." *Scientific American* (November 1989): 30–33.

Jennings, Charles. "Reflections on Transparent Motion." *Nature* 373 (February 16, 1995): 563.

Kaas, Jon H. "Vision Without Awareness." *Nature* 373 (January 19, 1995): 195.

Kalin, Ned H. "The Neurobiology of Fear." *Scientific American* (May 1993): 94–101.

Kandel, Eric R., and Robert D. Hawkins. "The Biological Basis of Learning and Individuality." *Scientific American* 267 (September 1992): 78.

Karni, Avi, et al. "Dependence on REM Sleep of Overnight Improvement of a Perceptual Skill." *Science* 265 (July 29, 1994): 679–82.

Kempler, Daniel, and Diana Van Lancker. "The Right Turn of Phrase." *Psychology Today* (April 1987): 20, 22.

Killheffer, Robert K.J. "The Consciousness Wars." *Omni* (October 1993): 50–59.

Kim, Seong-Gi, et al. "Functional Magnetic Resonance Imaging of Motor Cortex: Hemispheric Asymetry and Handedness." *Science* 261 (July 30, 1993): 615–17.

Kimura, Doreen. "Sex Differences in the Brain." *Scientific American* 267, no. 3 (September 1992): 118.

Kinoshita, June. "Dreams of a Rat." *Discover* (July 1992): 34–42.

_____. "Mapping the Mind." *New York Times Magazine* (October 18, 1992): 44–50, 52, 54.

_____. "Severed From Emotion." *Discover* (July 1992): 20.

Knowlton, Barbara J., and Larry R. Squire. "The Learning of Categories: Parallel Brain Systems for Item Memory and Category Knowledge." *Science* 262 (December 10, 1993): 1747–49.

Kolata, Gina. "Man's World, Woman's World? Brain Studies Point to Differences." *New York Times* (February 28, 1995): C1, C7.

_____. "Men and Women Use Brain Differently, Study Discovers." *New York Times* (February 16, 1995): A1, A22.

_____. "Mental Gymnastics." *New York Times Magazine* (October 6, 1991): 15–17, 42–43.

Kosslyn, Stephen M. "Aspects of a Cognitive Neuroscience of Mental Imagery." *Science* 240 (June 17, 1988): 1621–26.

LeDoux, Joseph E. "Emotion, Memory, and the Brain." *Scientific American* (June 1994): 50–58.

"Left-Brain Snow Job." *Science News* 136 (September 23, 1989): 204.

Lemonick, Michael D. "Glimpses of the Mind." *Time* (July 17, 1995): 44–52.

"Less Invasive Brain Imaging in Humans." *Science News* 145 (January 15, 1994): 47.

Lewin, Roger. "Refined Speech the Key to Being Thoroughly Human?" *Science* 236 (May 8, 1987): 670.

_____. "Seeking Hidden Messages in Stone Tool Technology." *Science* 236 (May 8, 1987): 669–70.

_____. "The Human Psyche Was Forged by Competition." *Science* 236 (May 8, 1987): 668–69.

_____. "What Makes Bigger Brains?" *Science* (June 30, 1989): 244.

Lindsay, Ronald M. "Neuron Saving Schemes." *Nature* 373 (January 26, 1995): 289–90.

Liversidge, Anthony. "Bacterial Consciousness: Why Spirochettes Think as We Do." *Omni* (October 1993): 10.

Llinas, Rodolfo. "Thorny Issues in Neurons." *Nature* 373 (January 12, 1995): 107–8.

"Looking at Inner Landscapes." *Economist* (July 3, 1995): 79–80.

"Mapping Chemical Changes in Brain." *USA Today* (February 1994): 3.

Marino, G. "Axon Acts: The Unbearable Likeness of Being." *Science News* 146 (August 27, 1994): 135.

Marshall, John C., and Peter W. Halligan. "Seeing the Forest But Only Half the Trees?" *Nature* 373 (February 9, 1995): 521–23.

McGinn, Colin. "Towards New Physics of Mind." A review of *Mental Reality*, by Galen Strawson. MIT Press, 1994. *Nature* 373 (February 2, 1995): 396.

McGuire, P. K., G. M. S. Shah, and R. M. Murray. "Increased Blood Flow in Broca's Area During Auditory Hallucinations in Schizophrenia." *Lancet* 342 (September 18, 1993): 703–6.

"Memory's Highways." *Psychology Today* (May 1992): 14.

Mestel, Rosie. "We're All Connected." *Discover* (January 1994): 88.

Miller, J. A. "The Brain's Behind Evolution's Drive." *Science News* 124 (August 13, 1983): 101.

Miller, Julie Ann. "It's All In the Timing." *BioScience* 43, no. 2 (February 1993): 80–81.

_____. "Putting It All Together." *BioScience* 43, no. 2 (February 1993): 84.

_____. "Sampling Locally in the Brain." *BioScience* 43, no. 2 (February 1993): 84–85.

_____. "The Brain's Rhyme and Reason." *BioScience* 43, no. 2 (February 1993): 82–83.

Miller, Kenneth D., Joseph B. Keller, and Michael P. Stryker. "Ocular Dominance Column Development: Analysis and Simulation." *Science* 245 (August 11, 1989): 605–15.

Mishkin, Mortimer and Tim Appenzeller. "The Anatomy of Memory." *Scientific American* (1987): 35–50.

Murphy, Decian G., et al. "X-Chromosome Effects on Female Brain: A Magnetic Resonance Imaging Study of Turner's Syndrome." *Lancet* 342 (November 13, 1993): 1197–1200.

"The Music of the Hemispheres." *Discover* (March 1994): 15.

"Musical Brains Pitch to the Left." *Science News* 147 (February 11, 1995): 88.

Nadis, Steve. "Kid's Brainpower: Use It or Lose It." *Technology Review* (November 1993): 19–20.

Naeye, Robert. "Magnetic Field Goal." *Discover* (June 1995): 23.

Nakanishi, Shigetada. "Molecular Diversity of Glutamate Receptors and Implications for Brain Function." *Science* 258 (October 23, 1992): 597–603.

"No . . . It's More Freudian." *Psychology Today* (October 1993): 25.

Nowak, Rachel. "Brain Center Linked to Perfect Pitch." *Science* 267 (February 3, 1995): 616.

O'Neill, Luke, Michael Murphy, and Richard B. Gallagher. "What Are We? Where Did We Come From? Where Are We Going?" *Science* (January 14, 1994): 181–83.

Ojemann, George A. "Cortical Organization of Language." *The Journal of Neuroscience* 11, no. 8 (August 1991): 2281–87.

Oliwenstein, Lori. "Monkey Think, Monkey Do." *Discover* (June 1989): 20.

Pellizzer, Giusseppe, et al. "Motor Control Activity in a Context-Recall Task" *Science* 269 (August 4, 1995): 702–707.

Pennisi, Elizabeth. "Grammar Skills Best Learned When Young." *Science News* 142 (November 28, 1992): 383.

_____. "Grunts Prep Babies for Talking." *Science News* 145 (March 5, 1994): 159.

_____. "Is This the Way Bobby Fischer Does It?" *Science News* (May 21, 1994): 327.

_____. "One Team, Two Clues in Alzheimer's Puzzle." *Science News* 146 (November 12, 1994): 308–9.

_____. "Quick, Easy Imaging of Brain Function." *Science News* 145 (March 5, 1994): 159.

_____. "Seeing and Controlling Chaos in the Brain." *Science News* 146 (August 27, 1994): 134

_____. "Seeing Synapses: New Ways to Study Nerves." *Science News* 145 (February 26, 1994): 135.

Pinker, Steven. "Rules of Language." *Science* 253 (August 2, 1991): 530–34.

Porush, David. "A Short History of Consciousness." *Omni* (October 1993): 64, 110.

_____. "Finding God in the Three-Pound Universe: The Neuroscience of Transcendence." *Omni* (October 1993): 60–70.

Posner, Michael I., et al. "Localization of Cognitive Operations in the Human Brain." *Science* 240 (June 17, 1988): 1627–31.

Posner, Michael. "Modulation by Instruction." *Nature* 373 (January 19, 1995): 198–99.

Raeburn, Paul. "Reverse Engineering the Human Brain." *Technology Review* (November 1993): 10–11.

Raichle, Marcus. "Images of the Mind: Studies With Modern Imaging Techniques." In *Annual Review of Psychology*, edited by Lyman W. Porter and Mark R. Rosenzweig. Palo Alto, Calif: Annual Reviews, Inc., 1994, 333–56.

————., et al. "Practice-related Changes in Human Brain Functional Anatomy During Nonmotor Learning." *Cerebral Cortex* (January 1994): 8–26.

————. "Visualizing the Mind." *Scientific American* (April 1994): 58–64.

Ramachandran, V. S., and S. Cobb. "Visual Attention Modulates Metacontrast Masking." *Nature* 373 (January 5, 1995): 66–68.

Rapoport, Judith. "The Biology of Obsessions and Compulsions." *Scientific American* (March 1989): 82–89.

Riccio, Cynthia A., et al. "Neurological Basis of Attention Deficit Hyperactivity Disorder." *Exceptional Children* 60, no. 2 (1993): 118–24.

Richardson, Sarah. "The Brain-Boosting Sex Hormone." *Discover* (April 1994): 30–31.

Riska, Bruce, and William R. Atcheley. "Genetics of Growth Predict Patterns of Brain-Size Evolution." *Science* 229 (August 16, 1985): 668–71.

Rugg, Michael. "La Différence Vive." *Nature* 373 (February 16, 1995): 561–652.

Sapolsky, Robert. "How Big is Yours?" *Discover* (March 1992): 40–43.

Schlaug, Gottfried, et al. "In Vivo Evidence of Structural Brain Asymmetry in Musicians." *Science* 267 (February 3, 1995): 900–1.

Seeking the Source of Emotions." *Science News* 138 (September 9, 1990): 175.

Sejnowski, Terence J. "Models of Vision." A Review of "Computational Models of Visual Processing," by Michael S. Landy and J. Anthony Movshon. *Science* 257 (July 31, 1992): 687–88.

Selkoe, Dennis J. "Aging Brain, Aging Mind." *Scientific American* 267, no. 3 (September 1992): 134.

Service, Robert F. "Making Modular Memories." *Science* 260 (June 25, 1993): 1876.

————. "New Alzheimer's Gene Found." *Science* 268 (June 30, 1995): 1845–46.

Shatz, Carla J. "Dividing Up the Neocortex." *Science* 258 (October 9, 1992): 237–38.

————. "The Developing Brain." *Scientific American* 267, no. 3 (September 1992): 60.

Shaywitz, Bennett A., et al. "Sex Differences in the Functional Organization of the Brain for Language." *Nature* 373 (February 16, 1995): 607–9.

Simon, C. "Motion Sickness is Partly in the Brain." *Science News* 124 (November 26, 1983): 342.

Simons, Elwin L. "Human Origins." *Science* 245 (September 22, 1989): 1343–50.

Skolnick, Andrew A. "New MRI Techniques Allow Noninvasive Peek Inside the Thinking Human Brain." *Journal of the American Medical Association* 268, no. 11 (September 16, 1992): 1387–88.

Snyder, Abraham Z., et al. "Scalp Electrical Potentials Reflect Regional Cerebral Blood Flow Responses During Processing of Written Words." *Proceedings. National Academy of Sciences* 92 (1995): 2365.

Squire, Larry R., B. Knowlton, and G. Musen. "The Structure and Organization of Memory." In *Annual Review of Psychology,* edited by Lyman W. Porter and Mark R. Rosenzweig. Palo Alto, Calif: Annual Reviews, Inc., 1993, 453–95.

Steriade, Mircea, David A. McCormick, and Terrence J. Sejnowski. "Thalamocortical Oscillations in the Sleeping and Aroused Brain." *Science* 262 (October 29, 1993): 679–88.

Stipp, David. "Partial Recall: Amnesia Studies Show Brain Can Be Taught at Subconscious Level." *Wall Street Journal* (October 5, 1993): A1, A4.

Stone, Richard. "Molecular 'Surgery' for Brain Tumors." *Science* 256 (June 12, 1992): 1513.

Strobel, Gabrielle. "Different Memories Go Different Places." *Science News* 144 (November 27, 1993): 367

––––––. "Pugnacious Mice Lack Serotonin Receptor." *Science News* 144 (November 27, 1993): 367.

––––––. "Young Brain Sports Marijuana Receptors." *Science News* 144 (November 27, 1993): 367.

"Study Finds Men's Brains Deteriorate at Greater Rate." *New York Times* (April 2, 1993): C2.

"The Stuff Memories Are Made Of." *U.S. News & World Report* (November 13, 1989): 16–17.

Suplee, Curt. "Sexes Shown to Think Differently: In Rhyming Task, Women Use Both Sides of the Brain, Men Just the Left." *Washington Post* (February 16, 1995): A1, A10.

Tank, D. W., A. Gelperin, and D. Kleinfeld. "Odors, Oscillations, and Waves: Does It All Compute?" *Science* 265 (September 23, 1994): 1819–20.

"Tracking the Brain's Language Streams." *Science News* 143 (June 19, 1993): 399.

Travis, J. "Brain Scans Hint Why Elderly Forget Faces." *Science News 148* (July 15, 1995): 36.

_____. "Do Brain Cells Run Out of Gas?" *Science News 148* (August 5, 1995): 84.

Trotter, Bob. "Better Memory Through Chemistry." *American Health* (April 1991): 12.

Vaadia, E., et al. "Dynamics of Neuronal Interaction in Monkey Cortex in Relation to Behavioural Events." *Nature* 373 (February 9, 1995): 515–18.

Waddington, John L. "Sight and Insight: 'Visualisation' of Auditory Hallucinations in Schizophrenia?" *Lancet* 342 (September 18, 1993): 692–93.

Waldolz, Michael. "Panic Pathway: Study of Fear Shows Emotions Can Alter 'Wiring' of the Brain." *Wall Street Journal* (September 29, 1993): A1, A12.

Weiss, Rick. "Ferrets, Looking Loudly, Hear the Light." *Science News* 138 (December 10, 1988): 374.

_____. "Shadows of Thoughts Revealed." *Science News* 138 (November 10, 1990): 297.

Whittington, Miles A., et al. "Synchronized Oscillations in Interneuron Networks Driven by Metabrotropic Glutamate Receptor Activation." *Nature* 373 (February 16, 1995): 612–15.

Willis, Jr., William D. "Cold, Pain and the Brain." *Nature* 373 (January 5, 1995): 19–20.

Wilson, Matthew A. and Bruce L. McNaughton. "Reactivation of Hippocampal Ensemble Memories During Sleep." *Science* 265 (July 29, 1994): 676–79.

_____. "Dynamics of the Hippocampal Ensemble Code for Space." *Science* 261 (August 20, 1991): 1055–58.

"A Window on the Brain." *Discover* (July 1992): 16.

Winslow, Ron. "A Nose Knows Secrets of Brain and Nerve Cells." *Wall Street Journal* (October 6, 1993): B1, B6.

Zeki, Semir. "The Visual Image in Mind and Brain." *Scientific American* 267 (September 1992): 68.

INDEX